XENO

David K.C. Cooper

MD . PhD . FRCS

Robert P. Lanza

MD

X E N O

**the promise of transplanting
animal organs into humans**

○ ○ ○ ○ ○ ○ ○ ○ ○ ○ ○ ○ ○ ○ ○ ○

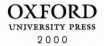
OXFORD
UNIVERSITY PRESS
2000

OXFORD
UNIVERSITY PRESS

Oxford   New York
Athens   Auckland   Bangkok   Bogotá   Buenos Aires   Calcutta
Cape Town   Chennai   Dar es Salaam   Delhi   Florence   Hong Kong   Istanbul
Karachi   Kuala Lumpur   Madrid   Melbourne   Mexico City   Mumbai
Nairobi   Paris   São Paulo   Singapore   Taipei   Tokyo   Toronto   Warsaw

and associated companies in

Berlin   Ibadan

Published by Oxford University Press, Inc.
198 Madison Avenue, New York, New York 10016

Oxford is a registered trademark of Oxford University Press

Library of Congess Cataloging-in-Publication Data
Cooper, D.K.C. (David K.C.), 1939–
Xeno : the promise of transplanting animal organs into humans /
by David K.C. Cooper, Robert P. Lanza.
Includes bibliographical references and index.
ISBN 0–19–512833–8
1. Transplantation of organs, tissues, etc.—Moral and ethical
aspects.   2. Xenografts—Moral and ethical aspects.
3. Transplantation immunology.   I. Lanza, R.P. (Robert Paul),
1956–   . II. Title.
RD120.7.C665 2000 617.9'5—dc21 99–14437

9   8   7   6   5   4   3   2   1

Printed in the United States of America
on acid free paper

To my mother, who, sadly, died the week
this manuscript was completed
D K C C

THE CREATURES outside looked from pig to man, and from man to pig, and from pig to man again; but already it was impossible to say which was which.

—GEORGE ORWELL (ANIMAL FARM)

THERE CAN BE few subjects in biomedicine more interesting or more challenging than xenotransplantation. The renewed interest has reached fever pitch. The stakes are high, the list of stakeholders is large, there are many unknowns, and the field is evolving rapidly.

—ABDUL DAAR, PROFESSOR OF SURGERY

IT HAS BECOME commonplace, such is the pace of innovation and development in medicine, that "frontiers" are identified, only to be crossed and assimilated with ease into the medical map in what seems like the blink of an eye. Thus, to describe xenotransplantation as a frontier in medical science is to invite a raised eyebrow on the world-weary and to risk relegating it to the status of this season's fashion. Yet, for once, the description may be apt.

—IAN KENNEDY, PROFESSOR OF MEDICAL LAW AND ETHICS
AND CHAIRMAN, UK ADVISORY GROUP ON THE ETHICS OF XENOTRANSPLANTATION

THE PROSPECTS for the applicability of routinely available grafts without the horrendous ethical, logistic, and economic problems that are entailed in the current use of human tissue for graft purposes are easy to underestimate. We don't really have an adequate vision of the way in which remedial medicine would be totally transformed if organs could be replaced at will, at fairly low cost, and with a high degree of reliability and a minimum of side effects.

—JOSHUA LEDERBERG, NOBEL LAUREATE

contents

Robin Cook, M.D.

An appreciation

o o o We are extremely grateful to Robin Cook for agreeing to contribute the foreword to this book. Before turning his talents toward writing novels, Robin Cook had a distinguished medical career. After graduating *summa cum laude* from Wesleyan University, he earned his medical degree from Columbia College of Physicians and Surgeons in New York. Training in surgery followed, at which time he was drafted into the U.S. Navy, where he attended submarine and diving schools. He subsequently undertook a second residency, this time in ophthalmology at Harvard. Upon its completion, he practiced as an eye surgeon and accepted a clinical teaching position at the prestigious Massachusetts Eye and Ear Infirmary of Harvard Medical School.

Robin Cook is one of the most popular novelists of our time and has brought a range of social issues to the attention of millions. He is widely credited with inventing the medical-thriller genre with his book *Coma,* which addressed the issues of human organ donation at a time when most types of organ transplantation were not even established forms of medical therapy. Since then, he has written 18 best-sellers, which have been translated into some 50 languages and have sold over 100 million copies. Robin Cook's books have frequently involved topics that are at the cutting edge of medical science, including xenotransplantation in *Chromosome 6.* As a surgeon whose thoughts and imagination are so consistently at the forefront of medical science, we felt it fitting to invite him to contribute the foreword to *Xeno.*

David K. C. Cooper
Robert P. Lanza

foreword

by Robin Cook

○ ○ ○ "Come on, you guys," Lou pleaded. "Don't make me beg. What the hell is a xenograft?"

"It's when a transplant organ is taken from an animal of different species," Laurie said.

"You mean like that Baby Fae baboon heart fiasco 10 or 12 years ago?" Lou asked.

"Exactly," Laurie said.

"The new immunosuppressant drugs have brought xenografts back into the picture," Jack explained. "And with considerably more success than with Baby Fae."

The above quote, from my book *Chromosome 6*, indicates the very reason why I chose xenotransplantation as the basis of my story. As far as medical research is concerned, xenografts are very much back into the picture, and trials in human patients are already taking place.

Organ transplantation is one of the miracles of 20th-century medicine. With its success, however, has come tragedy. As a doctor, I know all too well that the demand for organ transplants far exceeds the supply of organs. Thousands of people die every year while waiting for donor organs. At the present time, clinical organ transplantation is limited largely to the use of organs retrieved from brain-dead (cadaveric) humans under less-than-ideal emergency conditions. Perhaps in the future, people with failing organs will have new ones fabricated in the laboratory by tissue engineering techniques. Laboratory-grown skin, bone, cartilage, and blood vessels are already being tested in patients. In fact, doctors at the University of Massachusetts recently used a piece of coral as a frame for bone cells to regenerate a patient's thumb after it had been severed in an industrial accident. Bioengineered body parts may eventually be able to restore vision to the blind, strengthen the bones of the weak, and replace organs and limbs. Fetuses may even grow in artificial wombs. In the meantime, however, xenotransplantation may be the only way to solve the problems inherent in the present system of dependency on human organs.

In this book, *Xeno*, the authors—both recognized experts in the field—delve into the many complex problems associated with animal-organ transplantation. They provide stimulating information on everything from the mechanism of organ rejection to the major impact xenotransplantation will have on health care economics. They look back into the intriguing history of xenotransplantation—from Serge Voronoff's chimpanzee testicular grafting operations in elderly men in the 1920s to the Baby Fae baboon heart transplant in the 1980s—and forward to the dramatic and exciting advances that can be anticipated within the next few years. However, many questions remain unanswered. Will the immunological hurdles of xenotransplantation be surmounted? Will a pig organ function adequately in the foreign environment of the human body? Could the transplantation of animal tissue create a public health hazard far greater than any previous "hot zone"? Does the genetically engineered or cloned "humanized" pig have any human legal rights? These are all interesting questions, and the authors address them, together with other scientific, social, and ethical issues, in a way that the lay individual will find both illuminating and readable.

My own medical thrillers have at times mirrored the activities of the medical and scientific communities so closely that readers have had a hard time determining when fact stops and fiction begins. *Coma*, written more than 20 years ago, highlighted problems that could develop in the field of human organ donation. The shortage of human donor organs continues to be an area of ethical concern for me. In this book, for example, David Cooper and Robert Lanza raise concerns about practices in China, where most transplanted organs come from executed prisoners. Human-rights activists claim that Chinese officials make money by taking whatever organs and tissues they require after an execution without the consent of the "donor." The possible retrieval of organs from political prisoners continues to be of particular concern.

I returned to the subject of organ transplantation several years later with *Blindsight* and, more recently, explored the world of xenotransplantation in *Chromosome 6*. This latter work represents a mixture of scientific fact and fiction that is only a step ahead of the real-life medical advances that are taking place today and which form the subject matter of *Xeno*. Although my novels were conceived as entertainment and can be categorized as fiction, they are based on hard medical and scientific facts and on my perception of medical science in the not-too-distant future. *Xeno* informs us that, in the field of xenotransplantation, the future has almost arrived.

Genetic engineering and cloning techniques—which were in the realm of science fiction not many years ago—today are being employed to "humanize" donor animals in several ways. The human recipient of an organ transplanted from such an animal will be tricked into recognizing the transplanted organ as "self" rather than "non-self." In short, the human body will think of the animal organ as human rather than foreign. Innovative new techniques and powerful drugs are becoming available to help overcome the remaining barriers to a limitless supply of spare body parts.

I share with the authors, and with others in the medical community, the opinion that these new and powerful techniques must be used responsibly. I also share their view that the use of monkeys and other nonhuman primates as organ donors is unjustified, not only because many of these species are endangered, but because of the much higher risk that a dangerous or even deadly virus could be inadvertently introduced not only into the organ recipient but into the human community at large. While xenotransplantation could eliminate the shortage of human donor organs, and thus render moot many of the associated ethical problems, it raises a new set of ethical concerns. This book provides information that will help society come to decisions on such matters.

Little in medicine, as in other human affairs, is a matter of black or white. For example, what happens when a doctor's responsibility to his patient—or a biotechnology company's responsibility to its investors—conflicts with his or her responsibilities to the public health at large? This ethical dilemma concerns and even scares me, and was a stimulus to my writing *Chromosome 6*. Great efforts are being made to ensure that the pigs being prepared today as the source of organs for humans are free from all possible bacteria and viruses. But this makes these animals very expensive to breed and maintain, and will place them beyond the financial reach of surgeons and patients in many of the world's poorer countries. Will it be only a matter of time before some of these frustrated surgeons and desperate patients take their chances with ordinary barnyard pigs as transplant donors? In fact, one of the authors of this book had just finished raising this same concern at a recent medical meeting when his co-panelist, Clark Colton, a distinguished professor at the Massachusetts Institute of Technology, took the microphone and added, "In Mandalay [in Southeast Asia] people keep a few chickens and a pig 'for those unexpected situations.' Xenotransplantation gives new meaning to this concept."

Xeno provides the intelligent and interested reader with an immense amount of clearly presented information, and is a welcome reminder that, despite the fact that things can (and sometimes do) go wrong in medicine, there are many doctors, scientists, and regulators working hard to ensure that they don't.

Robin Cook
Boston, Massachusetts

preface

The next great medical revolution?

o o o   Medicine is on the verge of its next great revolution—xeno-transplantation, or the transplantation of organs and tissues from animal species, such as the pig, to humans. The potential for this new field of medicine is simply enormous. Indeed, clinical trials are already taking place in patients using baboon cells for the treatment of AIDS, pig cells for diabetes and Parkinson's disease, cow cells for intractable pain, and pig livers as a temporary bridge to human organ transplantation. However, it is the potential for the permanent replacement of vital organs that has the greatest potential for capturing our imagination. It is to this aim that most efforts are being directed.

Organ transplantation is one of the great success stories of the second half of the 20th century. Almost half a million people worldwide have received an organ transplant during the past 40 years. Indeed, it is its very success, resulting in the referral of ever-increasing numbers of patients, that has led to the present crisis in donor organ supply. Xenotransplantation would provide a solution not only to the number of transplants that could be performed but also to other problems inherent in the present system of dependency on human organs. (*Xenos,* by the way, is Greek for "foreign" or "strange.")

The need for a limitless source of organs and tissues is immense, and the reasons for the great increase in research activity in xenotransplantation during the past 10 years can readily be appreciated. But are these endeavors likely to be successful? Or will we be perpetually faced by the prediction made by one cynical surgeon some 20 years ago, who said: "The future of transplantation is xenotransplantation. And always will be!"

This volume highlights the considerable progress that has been made. We have begun to understand the very real differences between the rejection of a transplanted animal organ and that of a human organ. This understanding has enabled new treatment options to be devised that increase our ability to modify the recipient's immune attack on the transplanted organ. The advent of genetic engineering and cloning techniques offers the prospect of donor organs that are protected from destruction by the human host. There is even work in progress aimed at inducing the human recipient to accept an animal organ without the need for immunosuppressive drug therapy.

The current wave of optimism in laboratories worldwide, however, will almost certainly be tempered by disappointment and setbacks. We shall probably look back and recognize the truth of the words of British transplant pioneer Sir Roy Calne, who fairly recently predicted that the use of animal organs in transplant patients "is just around the corner. But it may be a very long corner!" Nevertheless, the current ever-quickening pace of advance in biotechnology and drug development encourages us to believe that the inherent problems will be overcome, perhaps by the early years of the next century.

Having made that (perhaps rash) prediction, we are reminded of that made by no less an authority than British Nobel laureate Sir Peter Medawar, who in 1969 said: "We shall solve the problem by using heterografts [animal organs] one day if we try hard enough, and maybe in less than 15 years." This was one occasion when the brilliant man was clearly wrong. If the "father of transplantation biology" can be proved so wrong, perhaps there is wisdom in these words: "Predictions are risky, especially about the future!" (attributed by xenotransplantation pioneer Keith Reemtsma to former U.S. vice president Dan Quayle).

But even if the science is proved successful, are we justified in proceeding with such a form of surgical therapy? In other words, is it ethical? Let us assume that it will be the pig—rather than the baboon or other nonhuman primate—that will be the donor of organs, a choice for which there are many good reasons. From the perspective of the pig, there is surely no difference in being slaughtered to provide food or donor organs for humans. From the perspective of the dying patient in urgent need of a donor organ, the potential risks would seem worth taking. To quote Peter Medawar again: "One can be as philosophical as you like about the ethics of transplantation. The fact of the matter is, people would rather be alive than dead." Equally, this can be said of xenotransplantation.

However, other concerns have to be considered before we advance from the laboratory to the treatment of patients—a step that the Massachusetts General Hospital Xenotransplantation Advisory Committee has said will be a "historic event." These largely address the potential risk that pig viruses may be transferred from the transplanted organ into the human patient, and then spread to other members of the community, leading to an AIDS-like epidemic of infection. This possibility is currently under intense investigation and requires a definitive answer before medical science can make this next "giant leap for mankind."

The need for xenotransplantation is clear, its feasibility likely, and if it is carried out with due regulation and adequate safeguards, it would appear acceptable from an ethical perspective. The potential benefits are absolutely immense, and it could prove to be the next great medical revolution. We must therefore be positive in our approach to the hurdles that remain. As George Bernard Shaw wrote in his play *Back to Methuselah*: "You see things; and you say 'Why?' But I dream things that never were; and I say 'Why not?' "

David K. C. Cooper
Robert P. Lanza

acknowledgments

o o o   We express our gratitude to Robin Cook for contributing the foreword to this book. We also thank the many colleagues and friends in the medical and scientific communities who have kindly read and advised on parts of this book. Particular thanks go to Patrick Aebischer, Tony d'Apice, Michel Awwad, Leo Buhler, Albert Edge, Roger Evans, Jay Fishman, Julia Greenstein, Claus Hammer, Robert Hawley, Joren Madsen, Clive Patience, David Sachs, Mauro Sandrin, Megan Sykes, Aron Thall, and Lindsay Williams. We are also deeply indebted to Crystal Taylor of CompOne Services in Oklahoma, who has so expertly typed and retyped the manuscript. Several of the illustrations were prepared by Jenny Kukielski of Earls Colne in the United Kingdom, to whom we extend our thanks. Finally, we appreciate the editorial assistance we have received from Kirk Jensen, Susan Day, and their colleagues at Oxford University Press.

David K. C. Cooper
Robert P. Lanza

XENO

chapter 1

The End of the Night Shift

Organ transplantation today and tomorrow

The Future ○ ○ ○

Imagine this scenario. It is 4:00 A.M. near St. Louis, Missouri. A surgeon—a man in his early 40s—arrives for work. It is his daily routine. He parks his car and enters the building. He changes into green scrubs, exchanges his shoes for white clogs, puts on a cap and mask, and walks through into the scrub-up area, where his colleague, a woman of about the same age, is already scrubbing her hands with disinfectant. With their clean hands held out at shoulder height to ensure they are not contaminated by contact with their bodies, they carefully back through the door and enter the gleaming, spotlessly clean operating room. The scrub nurse, already gloved and gowned, hands them sterile towels, and they dry their hands and arms. She helps them into gowns and holds open surgical rubber gloves, into which they insert their hands.

The donor is already on the operating table, skin thoroughly cleaned with iodine, sterile drapes covering all but the chest and abdomen. The surgeons are greeted cordially by the anesthesiologist, standing at the head of the table, who is closely monitoring the sleeping donor's blood pressure and other vital signs. Three operating-room technicians, who have helped prepare the donor for the surgeons, are ready to assist with the retrieval of organs. Bottles of organ preservation fluid hang from stainless steel stands, and polystyrene boxes filled with ice line one wall.

The male surgeon deftly opens the donor's chest while his female colleague makes an incision the whole length of the abdomen. With two assistants, they work diligently for almost an hour, isolating the heart, lungs, liver, kidneys, and pancreas from the surrounding tissues. Finally, they are ready to stop the heart and excise the organs. Ice-cold solutions are infused into all of the selected organs. The heart stops instantly. The lungs, liver, kidneys, and pancreas become ghostly white as the blood is washed out of even the tiniest capillaries and their metabolism virtually ceases. Ice is packed around the organs to cool them further.

The heart is the first organ to be removed from the body. It is inspected for any anatomical abnormalities, then placed in a plastic bag containing cold saline and packed in a box of ice. The lungs soon follow, then the liver, kidneys, and pancreas, each sequestered individually in boxes of ice. Before the surgeons even take off their gloves, the polystyrene boxes have been hurried out of the building to a waiting van. Thirty minutes later, they are safely at the airport, the heart and liver bound for Omaha, the lungs and a kidney for Dallas, and the pancreas and remaining kidney for Denver.

The organs reach their various destinations in the holds of scheduled airliners, where they are rushed to the awaiting hospitals. Surgical teams already have the recipients prepared, and the organs are transplanted. The periods that have elapsed since the organs were removed from the donor are less than four hours for the heart and lungs, and a little longer for the other organs. They all function well, and six more patients have cheated death and been given a new lease of life.

Back at the donor center, the two surgeons have repeated the procedure twice more that morning. By 2:00 P.M., their day's work is over, barring an emergency request for a heart or possibly a liver, though such requests are rare.

Similar operative procedures have taken place at several other donor centers strategically placed throughout North America, in Europe, Japan, and Australia. A total of 200 organs has been distributed to waiting patients in the United States alone that day. Two hundred more will be distributed the next day and, indeed, every working day throughout the year, totaling 50,000 a year. A similar number will be transplanted in the rest of the world.

How can this be, you ask? How can so many organ donors become available every day? How can the donor retrieval procedures and the transplant operations be scheduled and coordinated so easily during the course of the day? The answer, of course, is that the donors of the organs are not humans, but specially bred pigs. The donor centers are not hospitals, but veterinary institutions situated in farms where the pigs are bred and reared by the thousands. Donor organs are therefore available on a daily basis—indeed, whenever required—greatly facilitating the logistics of organ transplantation.

The Present o o o

Compare the above with the current scenario relating to organ donation, a field in which one of the authors of this book was personally and continuously involved as a heart and lung transplant surgeon for almost 20 years.

"Inevitably, the telephone rings when I have just fallen asleep after a long day's work. The local organ donor coordinator is on the line. She has identified a potential brain-dead donor at a local hospital—a 19-year-old man with a fatal gunshot wound to the head. The heart, which is the organ of interest to me, is beating well and is a good size and blood group match for a patient in our intensive care unit. After some questioning regarding blood pressure, heart rate, blood gases, serum potassium level, and so on, I conclude that the heart seems suitable for my patient. A final decision, however, will await the results of certain blood tests, which should be available within the next 60 minutes.

"Local colleagues have already accepted the kidneys and pancreas, and a transplant center in the adjoining state has accepted the liver. But again, their final decisions are dependent on the results of the blood tests, which with luck will exclude any infectious agents in the donor's blood, including the viruses that cause AIDS (HIV) and hepatitis. Unfortunately, the lungs are not suitable for donation; the young man vomited after being shot in the head—a not unusual occurrence—and inhaled the vomit, thus damaging the lungs. The coordinator and I tentatively agree on the time the donor operation will begin, about two hours hence.

"I replace the telephone receiver, but immediately lift it again to contact my own hospital coordinator. I give her instructions regarding the preparation of the potential recipient, a man in his late 40s who has been in severe heart failure, too sick to leave the hospital, for the past six weeks. There are a battery of tests that have to be carried out and a number of drugs to be administered before the transplant can begin. The coordinator will organize these and, in addition, will inform my various colleagues—assistant surgeon, anesthesiologist, nurses, heart-lung machine technician—to be available at the agreed time in our operating room.

"These two telephone conversations have taken about 30 minutes. I try to get a little sleep. I know that if the donor blood tests prove satisfactory, I shall be busy for the next 18 hours performing organ retrieval and heart transplantation and supervising the recovery of the patient, in addition to the following day's routine work. It is difficult, however, to get back to sleep, as my mind is now fully awake and active.

"I have just fallen asleep again when the donor coordinator calls back with the blood test results. Unfortunately, the donor is positive for hepatitis C, a virus that can cause serious liver disease. This places all of the potential recipients at some risk from acquiring the disease—an unpleasant, debilitating, and potentially fatal one. The liver transplant group has already decided not to use the liver.

"I mull over this problem in my head. If I choose not to use the organ, will my patient live for at least a few more days—maybe a week or two—until another donor heart is offered? Or will he deteriorate and die before the next heart becomes available? I clearly don't want to put him at risk for developing hepatitis, but I would accept the risk if I thought he was likely to die within the next few days.

"Even with years of experience behind me, such decisions are always difficult, especially when they have to be made quickly and in the middle of the night when perhaps I am not thinking as clearly as I would when fresh in the morning. I am always aware of the subtle influence on my decisions of the state of my body, which is telling me to stay in this nice warm bed with my wife and not expose myself to the cold of the night. At this moment, nothing seems more attractive than sleep. I force myself to ignore this seductive influence and do what is best for my patient.

"I tell the coordinator I need a few minutes to think. I take the opportunity to call my patient's cardiologist and discuss the matter with him. He reassures me that the patient is not likely to die during the next few days. The cardiologist, like me, is inclined to wait for a heart from a donor who is negative for hepatitis C. I call the donor coordinator and let her know our decision, then phone the hospital coordinator, who is not too pleased with me, as she will now have to cancel all of the arrangements she has just made.

"It is now two hours since the first call to me, and I try once again to get some sleep. It is still difficult to do so, however; despite my confidence only five minutes ago, I run over in my mind yet again whether or not we have made the right decision. Eventually, I fall into a deep sleep. Within minutes, the telephone rings again. This time the donor coordinator informs me of a pair of lungs being offered from a distant center—approximately 750 miles from us—for a patient on our lung transplant waiting list. After 30 minutes of questions and answers, during which time the coordinator calls back to the donor center for further information, I accept the lungs.

"Yet again I call my hospital coordinator, and we make plans to admit the potential recipient, who is waiting at home, and mobilize all of the operating room staff. The patient is a young woman with cystic fibrosis who, healthwise, is reaching the end of the road. She has been on our waiting list for almost two years and has been called in twice in recent weeks on false alarms. This may be her last chance.

"I get out of my warm bed, wash, dress, and drive to the airport, where the hired Lear jet and its two-man crew are waiting. It is a bumpy and uncomfortable flight, and we can see much lightning in the distance. An ambulance picks us up at the airport and drives us to the donor hospital. It is now 4:00 A.M. I immediately telephone my hospital coordinator. They are running late. The potential recipient has only just arrived from home, and so I have to delay retrieval of the donor lungs for at least 30 minutes. I relay this information to the other retrieval teams. It is greeted with the usual lack of enthusiasm for delays at this hour of the morning.

"I scrub and join the group at the operating table. The lungs look healthy and the blood gases are fine. I do what little preparation of the lungs is necessary at this time, and then ask my coordinator to check how my hospital colleagues are doing. Fortunately, they are progressing well. The patient has reached the operating room and they are ready to begin. As I do not anticipate being back with them for at least two hours, this should give them time to anesthetize the patient and open her chest.

"We go ahead with the retrieval of the organs [which is performed in exactly the same way as described earlier for the pig]. I finally get back to my own hospital at 7:30 A.M. and we proceed with the lung transplants. It has been a long night, and there is still a long day ahead."

The differences between these two scenarios—donor organ retrieval in the pig and in the brain-dead cadaveric human—are obvious. If pigs could donate organs to humans, the advantages include not only convenience for the surgical teams, a relatively minor point, but also highly important factors that may make the difference between life and death for the recipient of the organs. We shall discuss these in the next chapter.

chapter 2

Animal Attraction

Supply and demand in the world of organ transplantation

The Heart Patient ○ ○ ○

The 14-year-old boy clings to life in the intensive care unit. Only three weeks previously he had been a normal, healthy teenager attending high school. Then he was struck down by a bout of nausea and vomiting, accompanied by a slight fever, which his parents initially put down to something he had eaten. After three or four days, when he showed no improvement, he was taken to his doctor, a rural primary-care physician, who, to his everlasting credit, noted an irregular heartbeat. The young boy was admitted to the local hospital, and transferred from there to the nearest university medical center, where he was diagnosed as being in heart failure. Only one week had passed since he had last played basketball.

No definite cause for his heart failure could be found, which many might consider surprising in this day and age of advanced medical technology. But a lack of a confirmed diagnosis is unfortunately common with this condition, dilated cardiomyopathy—indeed, confirmation is a relative rarity. The disease is not confined to teenagers, but occurs in all age groups. It has many known causes—and even more unknown ones. In the case of this young boy, his clinical history suggested it was associated with a viral infection, and so he was diagnosed as suffering heart failure caused by a viral inflammation of the heart—viral myocarditis.

The disease is poorly understood, but the diagnosis was confirmed by the cardiologist, who passed a catheter down a vein in the neck into the heart and, with a small pair of forceps, took a small bite out of the muscle of the heart wall. A pathologist examined this biopsy under the microscope, and confirmed that it was indeed myocarditis.

Despite a course of treatment with corticosteroid drugs, the boy's heart failure steadily worsened, and within a few days doctors decided to add his name to the waiting list for a heart transplant. His deteriorating condition required support with intravenous drugs, which held him stable for only a few days. The cardiologist was forced to insert an intra-aortic balloon pump, which is a simple mechanical device that assisted his heart further. In this precarious situation, clinging to life, he awaits a donor organ.

The likelihood of one becoming available within the next few days is negligible, even though he is on the priority list. At 14 years of age, he is probably going to die. The only alternative is an artificial heart—or left ventricular assist device, as they are more correctly known—which would require his transfer to one of the relatively few centers where these are available. Such transportation, even by air ambulance and accompanied by a doctor and a paramedic, carries significant risks, and there is a real possibility that he would not survive the flight. Furthermore, the boy's chest may be too small to accommodate the available assist devices. The hospital staff decide that his best chance is to stay in the intensive care unit and hope that a heart becomes available before he dies.

The Harsh Statistics o o o

Although the statistics of organ supply and demand do not bring home to the reader the personal stories and personal tragedies that they represent, let us examine the present situation. In the United States, over 63,000 patients await an organ of one type or another (see Figure 2.1 and Table 2.1), and a new name is added to the waiting list every 18 minutes. And yet only about 17,000 organs (from approximately 6,000 brain-dead donors) will become available this year. A further 3,700 organs (such as a kidney or part of a liver) will be obtained from living donors, bringing the total number of organ transplants to over 20,000. Two-thirds of the waiting patients will therefore be forced to wait another year—unless they die in the interim. The *average* wait in the United States for a liver is well over one year (Table 2.2); for a kidney or for a heart and both lungs (as a single procedure) it is over two years. The discrepancy between the number of people waiting and the number of organs that become available is increasing by 10 to 15% annually (see Figure 2.1).

The situation is similar in Western Europe and Australasia. In the United

figure 2.1. *Total number of patients awaiting organ transplantation on June 2, 1999 (upper curve), and total number of actual transplant operations performed each year from 1988 through 1998 (lower curve) in the United States. The number of patients awaiting organ transplantation is steadily rising and during 1999 reached over 63,000, whereas the number of cadaveric organs available for transplantation is almost static and remains at approximately 17,000. (Data from UNOS.)*

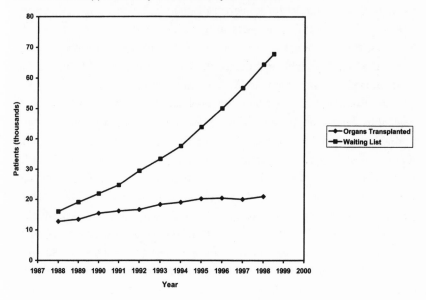

Kingdom more than 6,000 people await a donor organ at any one time, and yet only approximately 3,500 organs become available annually. In Western Europe as a whole, some 40,000 patients await a kidney, but only 5,000 brain-dead cadaveric donors are identified annually, providing 10,000 kidneys.

This imbalance in supply and demand has been made worse by two factors. One is a decrease in the number of accidental deaths—and thus in the number of donors—resulting from, for example, mandatory use of seat belts in automobiles and crash helmets when riding a motorcycle, together with laws outlawing drinking and driving and lowering speed limits. The other factor is the relative failure of health education programs, which has led to an increase in the number of potential transplant recipients; for example, smoking, alcoholism, and consumption of animal fats, together with a population that is steadily growing older and is thus more disease-prone, have increased the number of individuals in need of heart or liver transplants.

Because of these factors, a significant percentage of people on organ transplant waiting lists die before a donor becomes available. This is especially the case with those awaiting a liver transplant, where no form of me-

table 2.1

Numbers of Patients on U.S. Waiting Lists in 1999[a] and Receiving Organ Transplants in 1997[b]

Organ	Number of Patients on U.S. Waiting Lists as of June 2, 1999	Number of U.S. Transplants Performed During 1997 Where Organ Was Obtained from a Brain-Dead Donor	Number of U.S. Transplants Performed During 1997 Where Organ (or Part of Organ) Was Obtained from a Living Donor	Total Number of U.S. Transplants Performed During 1997
Kidney	42,071	7,759	3,669	11,428
Liver	13,095	4,100	68	4,168
Pancreas (or Pancreas + Kidney)	2,317	1,055	6	1,061
Heart	4,277	2,292	0	2,292
Lung	3,299	911	17	928
Heart + Lungs	238	62	0	62
Intestine	119	65	2	67
Total	63,635	16,244	3,762	20,006

Source: United Network for Organ Sharing (UNOS).

[a] Data as of June 2, 1999.
[b] Data from UNOS Annual Report, 1998.

table 2.2

Median Waiting Time (in Days) for an
Organ Transplant for Patients Registered in
the United States in 1997[a]

Kidney	962[b]
Liver	477
Pancreas	281
Pancreas + Kidney	375
Heart	207
Lungs	567[c]
Heart + Lungs	740[c]
Intestine	NA

Source: United Network for Organ Sharing (UNOS) Annual Report, 1998.

[a] The last year for which data are available.
[b] Data for 1995. Among patients registered in 1996 and 1997, too few have been transplanted to make it possible to calculate the median waiting times.
[c] Data for 1996.
NA = Data not available.

chanical device is available to keep the patient alive (Table 2.3). Approximately 11 patients die in the United States every day while awaiting an organ—more than 4,000 per year, or 5% of those waiting for an organ. This figure has more than doubled in the past 10 years. For patients awaiting a heart and lungs, the percentage who die rises to above 15%. For those with a rapidly deteriorating heart or liver, of course, the mortality rate is much higher. Complicating the situation is the fact that some lung transplant surgeons believe that once a patient's disease has advanced so far that he or she can be kept alive only by a mechanical ventilator that pumps oxygen in and out of his or her lungs through a tube passed through the nose or mouth, the risks involved in lung transplantation have become too high to be acceptable.

The Lung Patient ○ ○ ○

In another city, a 55-year-old woman with long-standing lung disease sits at home in her favorite armchair watching television, a portable oxygen cylinder by her chair. She has been totally dependent on oxygen for almost two years and has been awaiting a lung transplant for more than 12 months. As there

table 2.3

*Number of Deaths of Patients Awaiting an Organ Transplant in the
United States in 1997*[a]

Organ	Patients	Deaths	% Who Died
Kidney	49,762	2,009	4.0
Liver	15,061	1,129	7.5
Pancreas	656	11	1.7
Pancreas + Kidney	2,654	120	4.5
Heart	7,298	774	10.6
Lung	4,056	409	10.1
Heart + Lungs	374	57	15.2
Intestine	NA	NA	NA
Total	79,679	4,327	5.4

Source: United Network for Organ Sharing (UNOS) Annual Report, 1998.

[a] Last year for which data are available.
NA = Data not available.

is no emergency status for patients awaiting lung transplantation, the likelihood is that she will wait at least another six months before her name reaches the top of the waiting list. In the meantime, she is restricted to her home, with the occasional visit to her daughter whenever her son-in-law can find time to transport her in his car. But these visits tax her to the limit, and so she now undertakes them only when the confines of her house become unbearable.

Every personal or household chore, which to those of us in good health are trivial routines and go almost unnoticed, is for her a major undertaking. In the morning it takes her more than an hour to wash her face, clean her teeth, and comb her hair, every stroke of the brush or comb being followed by a minute's rest while she sucks in the life-giving oxygen. A further 45 minutes is needed to put on a few loose-fitting clothes. Then she must rest until lunchtime. Preparing herself a sandwich is the most she can do during the middle of the day. Then it is back to the chair, where she sleeps for an hour or two. In the evening, preparing a little meal is a protracted and energy-sapping, almost painful undertaking. After watching television for a couple of hours, she retires—slowly—to bed, exhausted from her day. Bathing is out of the question, and she must do the best she can sitting beside her bathroom sink.

Her husband died some years ago from a heart attack, and so she has no help in the home. Her daughter does the little shopping that she requires. A few visitors help to break the monotony of the day, but the demands of talking are so exhausting that she is equally pleased to see them go. Her only hope is a lung transplant, but donor lungs are among the organs most difficult to obtain. She has a greater than one in five chance that she will die before a lung becomes available to her.

Closing the Donor-Recipient Gap o o o

Every effort has been made both to encourage organ donation and to utilize those organs that become available. Elaborate organizations have developed throughout the Western world to ensure that potential donor organs are not wasted. In the United States, the United Network for Organ Sharing (UNOS) coordinates organ donation throughout the country, and similar networks exist throughout Europe and elsewhere. More than half of the states in the United States have passed laws requiring hospitals to raise the possibility of organ donation with the relatives of dying patients. Some European countries have introduced a "presumed consent" law, whereby a potential donor can be considered to have consented to donation unless he registered an objection during his lifetime; however, few transplant centers will remove organs from a potential donor in the face of family opposition, even though this would be legal in such countries. And yet donor supply increasingly fails to meet the demand.

Every opportunity is taken to draw this need to the public's attention. Every celebrity who requires an organ transplant—be they actor, athlete, or politician—is given maximum publicity, and many run-of-the-mill organ transplants performed on ordinary people are still considered newsworthy in the recipient's hometown. The public's attention is continually being drawn to the never-satisfied need for donor organs, but this has not worked to increase supply.

In every country, there are definitely potential donors who are not being identified or from whose family consent cannot be obtained. In most of the Western world, between 10 and 20 of every million brain-dead individuals are donors. In Spain, however, the donor rate is approximately 30 per million, about double the figure elsewhere. This is not because more patients are suffering brain death in Spain, but is the result of a highly efficient system for identifying potential donors and for approaching their families. In almost every Spanish hospital, there is a doctor, nurse, or other individual who is paid to identify and "acquire" potential donors. (Financial incentives in the field of organ supply may be a more important factor than generally recognized, as discussed briefly in Chapter 15.) The Spanish estimate that even they lose 22% of potential donors, as the family fails to give permission for use of the organs.

But even if organ retrieval could be doubled in the United States—which for a number of reasons is unlikely to happen—supply would still be insufficient to meet the rapidly increasing demand. Careful estimates have been made of the total number of organs that would become available if *every* potential donor donated his or her organs for transplantation, and even then, the supply would not meet the demand. This is because in the majority of cases the cause of death or the mechanism of dying make the organs unsuitable for transplantation. For example, those dying of cancer risk transferring their disease, as do those suffering from widespread infection. Heart attacks, diabetes, and many other conditions can render organs diseased and unusable. In fact, it has been estimated that even of those dying in hospital, only 4% are suitable to be considered as potential organ donors. Thus if we continue to rely entirely on cadaveric human organs (that is, organs removed from brain-dead individuals), there seems to be no solution to the problem.

Living Donors ○ ○ ○

Enormous efforts have been made to utilize the organs of close living relatives of the potential recipient. This is most common when a relative donates a kidney to a family member. More recently, this concept has been extended to donation of part of a liver, particularly between parent and child. Even parts of lungs have been transplanted from parent to child on a small number of occasions.

Donations of kidneys from living donors unrelated by birth, such as spouses or close friends, is on the increase, although the advantage of close genetic match with the recipient is lost. Donation under such circumstances has to be monitored carefully to ensure that the donor has a close emotional relationship with the recipient. The donation must be freely given and altruistic, and in no way coerced. The operation on the donor, particularly removal of part of the liver or lung, is complex and time-consuming, and not without risk of complication. Although the loving parents, siblings, spouses, or friends who offer to donate an organ or organ part are to be commended, and, though this approach is being encouraged, it will unfortunately not solve the enormous problem of inadequate donor organ supply.

The Kidney Patient ○ ○ ○

In another town, before going to bed each night, the young mother takes the spigot out of the catheter that was surgically inserted into her abdominal cavity and is protruding from her stomach wall. She plugs in the infusion cannula from the dialysis solution. She has been doing this every night for five years. While she is asleep, the dialysis fluid will drip in and out and help replace the activity of her nonfunctioning kidneys. At first, the nightly ritual was a chore, and she slept poorly. Every time she moved, she was fearful of disconnecting the dialysis solution, which she did do on a number of occasions. However, over the years, she has adapted to the inconvenience and now sleeps fairly well.

But peritoneal dialysis is a poor substitute for normal kidneys. She remains anemic, with a lack of energy that makes life a mere shadow of its former self. Still, she is happy just to be alive; at least she can watch her little boy grow up.

Her name has been on the waiting list for a donor kidney for more than two years. She was called to the hospital on one occasion when the tissue match was perfect, but the transplant was canceled at the last minute, as the surgeon was not happy with the performance of the donor kidney. She patiently awaits a further call to the hospital, but it may be another year before this occurs.

Her husband has had to rush her to hospital on two occasions during the past year when the abdominal catheter became infected and she suffered severe abdominal pain and a high fever. Fortunately, treatment with intravenous antibiotics saved her life on each occasion, and both times she was temporarily transferred to hemodialysis—using an artificial kidney machine—to allow time for her peritoneal infection to resolve. This necessitated her visiting the hospital for six hours a day, three days a week, which disrupted her life even more.

Organ Brokers: The Ethical Dilemma ○ ○ ○

About 70,000 U.S. citizens develop kidney failure each year. The majority begin on some form of dialysis while they await a transplant. For a not insignificant number, however, the quality of life possible with dialysis deteriorates to the extent that they choose to discontinue this form of therapy even though they know that this will mean death; renowned writer James Michener was one such person. The fortunate will eventually receive a kidney transplant.

But consider the plight of a patient in renal failure in a country where, because donation of organs after death is not part of the culture of the community, the organ shortage is extreme. This is the case in many countries in Asia. Even if such a person could afford to travel to Europe or North America and live there while awaiting a transplant, most of these countries severely restrict the number of organs that can be transplanted into nonresidents or foreigners.

Some wealthy individuals in this situation have found a way around their dilemma with the help of brokers who can arrange for a poverty-stricken man or woman to agree to give up a kidney—for a price. We may see this as an unethical enticement or even a form of coercion, but many such paid donors will quickly offer a "superfluous" organ—one of a pair, such as a kidney—for a sum that to them may represent untold wealth.

One could argue that there is nothing inherently wrong in such an arrangement as long as both recipient and donor are given excellent medical care. After all, if we accept that an unrelated friend can donate a kidney (without financial reward), then we must believe that, with Western medicine, there is insignificant risk to the health of the donor, either short-term or long-term. The only difference in this case is that we are considering whether the donor can be paid—a practice called "rewarded gifting."

Such practices have been officially outlawed in many countries, but not all, and it is not within the scope of this book to delve into a lengthy discussion of the pros and cons, and of the ethics, of such brokered arrangements. Indeed, it could be argued that relatively affluent members of the Western world are not in a position to pass judgment on the actions of either the recipient or the donor in such cases. How can we fully understand or appreciate the frustrations and fear of a patient dying of kidney disease in, for example, India or the Middle East, where few or no cadaveric organs are available? How can we presume to judge such a donor when most of us have no inkling of what the life of a man or woman living in such abject poverty is like?

Unfortunately, the brokered system as it currently exists in some parts of the world is open to abuse—and not only of the donor. Neither donor nor recipient may be given acceptable post-transplant medical care. After the first few days, the donor is medically abandoned. And the same fate may await the recipient once he has returned to his region or country of origin. At worst, the donor is paid inadequately or cheated of his money, the recipient pays an extortionate price, and only the broker and surgeon profit from the procedure. This is just one example of the extreme ethical problems that can arise purely as a result of the worldwide inadequate supply of human donor organs for transplantation.

The Liver Patient o o o

A young man walks into a hospital late one morning, jaundiced and weak but otherwise relatively well. Within hours, however, he deteriorates dramatically and by midnight has lost consciousness. Transfer to the intensive care unit does little to improve him; his "fulminant liver failure" is believed to be due to a hepatitis virus, which has rapidly overwhelmed his body. There is no alternative to a transplant, and he is immediately placed at the top of the waiting list for a donated liver. If he remains unconscious for more than a day or two, the toxins that the liver fails to remove from his blood will damage his brain permanently, and it is unlikely he will recover.

A less-than-ideal liver becomes available the following day. Its function is poor, and under normal circumstances, the surgeon would not accept it. But the young man's plight is desperate and the surgeon takes the chance. The transplanted liver never functions satisfactorily, and within hours, the patient's name is placed back on the waiting list for a second transplant. No new liver becomes available, and he dies the following day.

The four brief clinical histories outlined above are typical of many patients on organ transplant waiting lists throughout the Western world. Kidney patients wait seemingly forever, lung patients cling to life for months or years, some not surviving long enough to obtain the "gift of life," and heart and liver patients may die rapidly because of the inadequacy of donor supply.

The Real Extent of the Problem ○ ○ ○

Despite the limitations and problems relating to the transplantation of organs from cadaveric and living donors in North America, Western Europe, and Australia, at least the possibility exists in such places. But for the vast majority of the world's population, transplanting human organs is either unthinkable or impossible.

In many countries, removal of organs from brain-dead subjects is still illegal or culturally unacceptable, and organ transplantation remains minimal. In Japan, for example, where the advanced surgical technology and expertise to carry out organ transplantation are in place, cadaveric organ transplantation is still very rarely performed. If animals could be used as organ donors, the situation would change dramatically. From the mere handful of organ transplants from related, living donors performed each year—mainly kidney and, to a lesser extent, partial liver transplants—transplantation would rapidly expand to the numbers seen in the Western world.

India, the Middle East, and southeast Asia are other regions where organ transplantation remains minimal, but where the demand is considerable. In India alone, an estimated 100,000 new patients present with kidney failure each year. In many of these countries there are centers with the facilities and expertise to perform organ transplantation—but, because of legal or cultural barriers, there are few or no donors.

Even in the Western world, the official numbers for those awaiting organ transplantation are not fully representative of the real situation. One statistic alone illustrates this point. Although there are approximately 40,000 patients officially awaiting a kidney transplant in the United States (Table 2.1), there are almost 250,000 people on regular dialysis, and 70,000 new patients diagnosed with renal failure each year. This suggests to Alan Hull, of the National Kidney Foundation, that should all 40,000 on the list suddenly receive transplants, there would very soon be another 40,000 names added to the waiting list. In the world as a whole, there are an estimated 700,000 patients on dialysis.

The Borderline Candidate o o o

From long personal experience we know that the limited availability of donors heavily influences the surgeon's decision whether to accept a patient to receive a transplanted organ. Any patient with a significant health condition that might adversely affect long-term survival following a heart transplant will most likely not be put on the waiting list for a donated heart. For example, someone with diabetes who has vascular disease not only in the heart but also in the arteries to the brain or to the legs is at higher risk for complications both at the time of the transplant and at all times in the future. Such a person's long-term outcome will almost certainly not be as good as that of a patient who does not have advanced diabetes. The surgeon's thinking is that he or she cannot afford to "waste" such a valuable resource as a donor heart on a patient whose chance of surviving 5 or 10 years after the transplant is considered significantly less than that of other patients.

Other such borderline candidates include those with disease of organs other than that to be transplanted. Someone with chronic bronchitis who needs a heart transplant is one such example, as is the patient with relatively minor coronary artery disease of the heart who needs a liver or lung transplant. The chronic bronchitic's impaired lung function will greatly complicate his postoperative recovery, and the patient with coronary disease is at risk of suffering a heart attack from the stress of a liver or lung transplant operation. In both cases, the concomitant condition may significantly impair the patient's long-term recovery. At worst, if the patient dies, the transplanted organ will have been wasted. At best, the organ will have been given to someone who may never be able to get maximum benefit from it. There are a host of other conditions that make a patient a less-than-ideal candidate.

Ironically, those who already have a transplanted organ that is now failing and requires replacement frequently find themselves in this borderline category. The immunosuppressive drugs they have been taking since they received their first organ graft may have resulted in complications such as high blood pressure, high blood cholesterol levels, osteoporosis (loss of bone strength), diabetes, malignant skin or internal cancers, poor kidney function (in those with other transplanted organs), and persistent or intermittent infection. Any of these, particularly when present in combination, can preclude a patient from receiving a second transplant. Since the first transplant, the patient's immune system has become accustomed to the transplanted organ, and relatively little immunosuppressive drug therapy is required to suppress the remaining immune response. Once the first organ is removed and a second organ transplanted, however, the patient is faced with a whole new batch of tissue antigens (in the new transplanted organ), which will stimulate his or her immune system to go into overdrive in an effort to destroy what it perceives as a new foreign invader.

To prevent rejection, much larger doses of drug therapy will now be required for at least several months until the body slowly adapts to this second transplanted organ. The increased drug therapy may well aggravate the existing complications. The failing kidneys may cease functioning altogether, necessitating dialysis. Malignant tumors—until now seemingly controlled—may spread rapidly. Infection may flare up again. Already weak bones may collapse altogether. Diabetes may be much more difficult to control. Blood pressure will go up, as will the serum cholesterol level. The attending physicians may therefore feel that the risks are so great that they cannot advise that a second valuable donor organ be given to this particular patient when there are so many first-time candidates waiting.

There are even those who think that each deserving patient should be given only one chance through transplantation, the idea being that, as with many scarce and highly sought-after commodities in the marketplace, fairness is best served with a strict rule of only one per "customer." This issue is likely to become more acute in the future. Already, some 20% of patients receiving donor livers and 10% of those receiving hearts are undergoing retransplant procedures, and this percentage will presumably rise steadily over the next decade as more and more transplant patients reach the limits of their first graft. The number of organs being allocated to "returning customers" is bound to increase, eating away further at this precious and restricted resource.

The practice of most fully utilizing available organs through a rigorous selection of candidates in whom the transplant is thought to stand the greatest chance of success can even extend to denying transplants to those who behave in ways that are likely to jeopardize their long-term survival. For example, an unintelligent, ill-disciplined, or frankly irresponsible patient may well not be able to cope with the demands of a complex immunosuppressive drug regimen unless he or she has excellent support from family or friends. If the family is equally unable or unwilling to master the drug regimen (and all the other aspects of the long-term care of an organ transplant recipient) or is uncaring and unsupportive, then the patient is almost certainly doomed. A patient who has demonstrated irresponsibility in looking after a first trans-planted organ—and especially if he or she has lost the organ as a result—will almost certainly not be considered a good candidate for receiving a sec-ond organ. Is it ethically correct for a medical team to perform an organ transplant in such a patient, where there is a real risk of the organ being rejected or the patient dying from infection simply because he or she is not taking the drugs correctly? This is a particularly pertinent question when there are hundreds of other patients who could have benefited from that priceless resource. Nothing is more frustrating for members of the surgical team than to lose a patient for such an unnecessary reason.

(There is, of course, a risk that members of the transplant team will be influenced by an assumption, possibly based on previous experience, that a person of a certain type or from a specific background will not do well after an organ transplant. Preconceptions regarding, for example, the poor, the mentally handicapped, and those from inner-city minority ethnic groups could bias the decision regarding acceptability for transplantation. Suffice it to say that most centers take great pains to ensure that the patient is assessed individually and not categorized on the basis of being a member of a specific social group.)

If the number of organs becoming available annually were unlimited, *all* of these borderline patients could be given the opportunity of a transplant despite the risk that they may not do as well as some others. At present, however, they compete with others for organs, and in many centers those who are considered to be less "competitive" are not even put on the waiting list but have to struggle with what alternative medical therapy may be avail-able. When members of the transplant team make difficult decisions of this nature, they have to accept that in the majority of cases they are condemning the patient to an early death. Distasteful as this may be, many physicians believe that such decisions currently have to be made in order to make the best use of the available donor organs. Indeed, is it fair to the donor or do-nor's family, who have made this incomparable gift, if that gift is not utilized as judiciously as possible? Surely the unwritten contract with the donor's family demands the greatest possible care in the allocation of the organ.

If there were an unlimited number of donor organs, the number of pa-tients put on waiting lists—certainly for hearts and lungs and probably for livers also—would most likely double in number. In our own experience, only approximately 50% of those referred for heart transplantation are accepted onto the waiting list at some centers. A few of those not selected do not have disease advanced enough to warrant transplantation, but the majority have factors that make them less "competitive" as candidates. Relatively few of these factors would unequivocally rule out the patient, but in the world of limited supply, where many are competing for the same resource, they are sufficient to weigh against these unfortunate people.

The Limited Potential of Artificial Organs ○ ○ ○

Certainly one possible alternative to a heart transplant is the use of an artificial organ such as an artificial heart or ventricular assist device. Although great progress has been made in this field in recent years, the number of patients in whom one of these devices has functioned for more than one year can almost be counted on the fingers of both hands. Even the most modern devices require the patient to wear a battery belt around his or her waist and to change the batteries every eight hours unless the device is plugged in to the mains. This restricts life considerably, to say the least, and there is no doubt that the quality of such life is not as good as in the patient with a well-functioning heart transplant.

Even though these devices are steadily being improved and will likely prove an option for some patients, it seems that it will be many years before a power source for such a device can be made small enough to be inserted into the patient, either under the skin or within the chest or abdominal cavity. When this can be achieved, then these devices may well prove strong competition to heart transplants. Unfortunately, it seems unlikely that we shall see this within our lifetimes.

For patients awaiting lung or liver transplants, however, there is really no alternative to a human or animal organ. Artificial lungs and livers are in extremely early stages of development, and there is no realistic prospect of any implantable mechanical device becoming available in the near future. Although artificial kidneys have been in use for 50 years, no device has been developed that can be implanted permanently into the patient, emphasizing the great bioengineering problems that this entails. In regard to liver, lung, and kidney replacement, therefore, xenotransplantation would appear to be our only option for the foreseeable future.

The Tip of the Iceberg ○ ○ ○

In summary, if unlimited organs were available to us, such as from a suitable animal, a conservative estimate would be that we would at least double the number of organ transplants performed annually in the Western world. In addition, we would open up the opportunity to receive an organ transplant for patients in many other countries where such an opportunity is not currently available. And yet even this enormous expansion is only the tip of the iceberg.

First, the patients we have discussed in this chapter form a relatively small proportion of the total number of patients who *might* benefit from organ transplantation if the number of donor organs were not limited and if the drug therapy currently required to prevent rejection could be further improved or reduced. For example, almost 3 million Americans suffer from congestive heart failure with a further 400,000 new cases being diagnosed annually; deaths related to this condition are estimated at over 250,000 each year. Obviously, not all of these would be transplant candidates. But under the circumstances outlined above, a proportion of them might well be considered for transplantation rather than be subjected to other surgical procedures, such as repeated operative attempts to improve the blood supply to the heart muscle. Similarly, there are almost certainly far more patients with chronic lung disease who might benefit from lung transplantation than are being formally assessed at the present time.

The situation with regard to patients with liver failure is probably even more critical. It is estimated that in the United States some 27,000 patients die annually from liver disease, some as a result of long-term disease and others because of acute, overwhelming hepatic failure. Of the latter, some 2,000 patients die from acute viral hepatitis. For a wide variety of reasons, including, occasionally, ignorance on the part of the physician caring for the patient, some of these patients are never referred to a liver transplant center. Someday in the future, most of them will be.

Another possibility is that xenotransplantation could be used to save a person who experiences a crisis such as a massive heart attack. Such a patient could receive an immediate and life-saving heart transplant rather than die within a few hours—if a donor organ were available. Indeed, in the words of Swedish transplant surgeon Carl Groth, xenotransplantation offers the prospect of "instant" organ transplantation that could save thousands of lives each year.

Unenvisioned possibilities

Pioneers of open heart surgery, now a routine procedure, have remarked that back in the 1950s, when the techniques for such surgery were being developed and refined, they had no concept of the way in which this field of surgery would expand. Most of them believed that they would continue to perform one or two such operations each week for the foreseeable future. The reality is that in some major centers ten or more open-heart operations are being carried out each *day*!

We believe that just as the early pioneers of open heart surgery in the 1950s did not envisage heart surgery on the scale it is performed today, the physicians of the 1990s do not envisage the role of xenotransplantation as it may be in 40 or 50 years' time. The ready availability of new organs to replace diseased ones will make it unnecessary for the average patient to endure inadequate medical therapy that provides a suboptimal quality of life.

The problem of diabetes

Around the world there are an estimated 140 million patients with diabetes, many of whom take insulin injections every day of their lives. The insulin they use has, until recently, been pig insulin, which works very efficiently in humans. Just think how much easier it would be for the patients if, instead of porcine insulin injections, they were able to receive a transplant of pig pancreatic islet cells, which are the cells that actually produce the insulin. Furthermore, despite regular insulin administration, many of today's diabetic patients develop complications, as this form of therapy rarely controls the patient's blood glucose levels as well as would be hoped. Successfully transplanted pancreatic islet cells would produce insulin exactly as and when the body required it, which might well prevent or at least reduce these complications.

The transplantation of the whole pancreas, a large gland in the abdomen that has several functions, is still relatively less common than transplantation of other organs, and like any organ transplant, it is a major surgical procedure not without risk. The injection of insulin-producing pancreatic islets (which are scattered throughout the pancreas and can be isolated from the other cells in the gland), however, is a relatively minor procedure. The islets can be injected under the capsule of the kidney or at some other site where they will continue to function despite being removed from their normal habitat.

Pig or cow islets are ideal for this purpose, unlike human islet cells. There are a number of reasons for this. It is difficult to extract islets from the pancreas and, in the process, there is considerable wastage of these cells. The islets from a large number of pancreases—perhaps four or more—may therefore be required for a single patient. The relatively small number of human pancreases that become available would in no way supply the needs of the enormous number of patients afflicted with diabetes. Furthermore, there is some advantage in using islets from fetal, rather than adult, pancreases, but obviously even more of these very small glands would be required to supply the needs of a single patient. Human fetuses will clearly never be available in the necessary numbers, even if removing their pancreases for such a purpose were considered ethically acceptable to the community. If islet transplantation is to become a realistic possibility in the treatment of the millions of patients with diabetes, there is no alternative to the use of islets from animal species.

Cellular replacement therapy

The transplantation of groups of cells (as in islet transplants), as opposed to whole organs, has immense potential. A large number of medical conditions are caused by the failure of cells to function satisfactorily, but the exact causes of these failures are frequently unknown to us. Such conditions are particularly common in relation to the brain and to the endocrine glands, glands such as the thyroid, adrenal, and pituitary glands (as well as the pancreatic islets) that secrete their hormone(s) directly into the blood (and not into another organ, such as the digestive glands that secrete into the gut). Such cellular failure might be overcome by transplantation of the appropriate pig tissues into the deficient human patient. This form of replacement therapy, however, will not be confined only to those hormones manufactured by the endocrine glands. For example, cell degeneration in the brain and nerves causes such widely differing disorders as Parkinson's, Alzheimer's, and Lou Gehrig's diseases. Maybe these also can be alleviated by the transplantation of the related tissues from an animal source, as we shall discuss later in this volume.

As the technology develops, replacement therapy using animal tissues and organs may expand beyond all current concepts. With regard to the transplantation of tissues and cells, as opposed to whole organs, it is possible that the advent of new technologies—the ability to clone human cells, for example—may obviate or reduce the need for animal cells. There may, however, be ethical and legal barriers that prevent human cell cloning, particularly if animal cells are demonstrated to be equally effective as a therapeutic option. Only time will tell which of the many options offered by modern biotechnological advances will prove to be the best. To quote Allen Ginsberg, "There is nothing to be learned from history anymore. We're in science fiction now."

chapter 3

From Icarus
to the First Heart Transplant

Man's early attempts to bridge the species gap

Paris, 1921: Sexual Rejuvenation by Xenografting ○ ○ ○

The surgeon cuts out the testicle from the anesthetized donor, carefully carries it into the adjacent room, slices it into six sections, and delicately inserts three sections into each testicle of the recipient. As soon as the operation is completed, the surgeon repeats the procedure in a second elderly man, this time using the donor's remaining testicle. Who would donate *two* testicles? One may desire to be altruistic and help one's fellow man, but surely this is taking things a bit too far!

If you haven't already guessed, the donor is, of course, an animal—on this occasion a baboon. The year is 1921. The scene is the prestigious Collège de France in Paris, and the surgeon is Russian emigré Serge Voronoff (Figure 3.1).

"Between the 12th of June, 1920, and October 15, 1923, I performed fifty-two testicular grafting operations. The graft, in one instance, was taken from man; in all other cases the grafts were obtained from apes." So begins Voronoff's remarkable book *Rejuvenation by Grafting*, published in 1925, in which he details his surgical experiences. Most of the recipients were elderly men. A typical example is one 74-year-old Englishman who "walked with difficulty, leaning on a stick.... His memory was bad, his intelligence slow and sluggish. He presented all the characteristics of the senile type. He had been sexually impotent for 12 years." Eight months after his surgery, how-

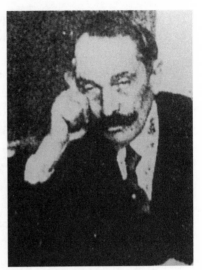

figure 3.1. *Serge Voronoff, the controversial Russian surgeon, who, working in Paris in the 1920s, carried out a large number of testicular transplants from chimpanzees and monkeys to elderly male patients. Many patients reported renewed vigor. (This photograph of a tired-looking Voronoff would suggest he might have benefited from this transplantation therapy himself!)*

ever, Voronoff was "stupified" at his patient's appearance. "The man was literally 15–20 years younger. His whole condition, physical, mental, and sexual, had undergone a radical change. The grafting had transformed a senile, impotent, pitiful old being into a vigorous man, in full possession of all his faculties." This "rejuvenation" continued for more than two years, until the patient died "during an attack of delirium tremens" from "intemperance," against which "unfortunately, the graft had no effect." Testicular transplants were clearly the Viagra of the 1920s—and more!

The response of the medical profession to Voronoff's testicular xeno-transplants was, to say the least, mixed, and usually highly skeptical. Jean Real, the French documentary film director, has researched Voronoff's work in some detail. He reports that each one of Voronoff's scientific presentations "threw the Académie des Sciences into turmoil." The public joined in the debate. "Many satirical newspapers and cabarets mocked the grafted men. The Folies Bergères even created a show around the subject. The whole of society laughed and the grafting of monkey 'balls' became a national joke. An ashtray representing a monkey protecting his private parts and with the text 'Non Voronoff, tu ne m'auras pas!' [No Voronoff, you won't get me!] was found on many cafe tables."

As no form of immunosuppressive drug therapy was given to any of his patients, it is exceedingly unlikely that any of the transplanted testicular tissue survived for more than a few days, if that. It is unlikely that the testicular grafts did any of his patients anything but psychological good. It is tempting, therefore, to label Voronoff a quack and a charlatan, but there is considerable evidence that he was a man whose vision exceeded the medical science of the time.

So convinced was he that higher monkeys would prove "a storehouse of spare parts for the human body" that he set up a farm on the French Riviera to breed monkeys imported from Africa, thus anticipating modern transplant surgeons—who are only now beginning to contemplate pig farms to provide organs for humans—by more than 70 years. Jean Real's research has also revealed the fact that in 1914 Voronoff carried out a bone graft—the first of many—from a chimpanzee to a French soldier wounded in the trenches during the First World War.

Voronoff was equally ambitious to promote transplants from human organ donors (allografts), and predicted that "in large towns in which fatal accidents are so frequent and so varied, patients waiting for organ transplantations would be sent to special hospitals to which any person dying from an accident would be transferred and, after thorough examination, his or her organs would be removed in order to be transplanted." Indeed, if luck had been on his side, Voronoff would have had the distinction of performing the world's first human kidney transplant; in 1928, while he was working in Paris, the authorities denied him permission to utilize the kidney of a criminal executed by guillotine who had donated his body to science. (The first human kidney transplant was therefore delayed until 1933, when Voronoff's compatriot, Voronoy, performed such a procedure in Russia.)

Daedalus and Icarus:
Xenotransplantation in Mythology ○ ○ ○

But Voronoff was by no means the first to contemplate transplanting organs from animals to humans, a subject that has intrigued man for as long as he has recorded his myths and history. According to contemporary xenotransplant pioneer Keith Reemtsma, whose tongue was firmly in his cheek, Daedalus, who grafted bird feathers to his arms, accomplished the first successful transplant across the species barrier. Legend has it that Daedalus escaped from his island prison in Crete and flew to the mainland of Greece. A similar experiment carried out by his son, Icarus, ended in disaster. After flying too close to the sun, Icarus is reported to have plunged into the sea, probably as the glue holding on his feathers melted! In his honor, the stretch of water in which he is alleged to have met his doom is now called the Icaran Sea. Keith Reemtsma suggests that this may be the first account of acute xenograft rejection (though he admits it appears more likely to be attributable to failure

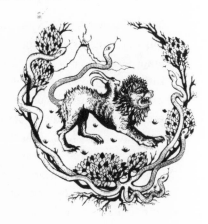

figure 3.2. *The mythological chimera, whose name has come to describe a human patient or animal in which native and donor cells survive together. (Illustration by Jenny Kukielski.)*

of a thermolabile adhesive). Nevertheless, he comments, "the overall 50% success rate achieved by this father-and-son team set an enviable record not matched for centuries."

Many of the fabulous beasts of mythology, such as the chimera (Figure 3.2), lamassu, griffon, hippocamp, and cockatrice, as well as creatures such as satyrs, centaurs, and mermaids, were clearly a combination of structures derived from several different species—in other words, they provided highly successful examples of xenotransplantation. Indeed, the chimera's name has been utilized in medical and scientific circles to describe an animal whose body consists of its own cells and cells from a donor.

The Earliest Years ○ ○ ○

Mythology and anecdote apart, xenotransplantation has been one of the holy grails of surgeons for centuries. Documented experimental work dates back more than 250 years and involved transplantation of glandular tissue, teeth, wings, and tails. The great British surgical investigator and anatomist John Hunter, working in London in the 18th century, carried out several attempts at xenotransplantation. His successful implantation of a human tooth into a cock's comb is well known in surgical circles. Although none of these experiments was of great lasting significance, they demonstrate the interest of surgical innovators in this field as far back as the 1700s.

Italy, 1628: blood transfusions from sheep to humans

Transfusions of animal blood to humans were documented as early as 1628 in Padua and soon after in London. In his excellent history of transplantation immunology, University of London immunologist Leslie Brent reports that this "therapy" was championed in the 1660s by a Professor Denis from France. Denis carried out several transfusions of sheep's blood in patients with varying conditions of ill health. After one such transfusion, a hitherto very sick patient is reported to have immediately leaped to his feet and engaged in vigorous activity, starting with slaughtering of the lamb that served as blood donor—which seems to be the height of ingratitude. Whatever immediate beneficial effect there might appear to have been from this highly incompatible transfusion might well be related to the fact that the poor patient had previously been subjected to "20 blood lettings" in an attempt to cure him.

In the 19th century, particularly in England, it became fashionable to transfuse those prone to violent outbursts, including wayward husbands and other troublemakers, with sheep's blood, in the belief that the sheep's docile personality would be transferred to the unfortunate recipient. One famous report referred to such therapy being administered to a scholarly fellow of one of the colleges of the University of Cambridge, who, despite his academic prowess, was wont to burst into violent tempers. Having survived the transfusion, he reputedly thanked his doctors for their attention and expressed a much-improved feeling of calmness and general well-being. We have also heard that sheep were used during the first World War as blood donors for wounded soldiers.

It is perhaps surprising that there are not many documented serious complications, as the sheep red blood cells would have been rapidly destroyed by human antibodies. This would almost certainly have been accompanied by fever, chills, transient jaundice, discolored urine, and possibly more serious complications, such as acute kidney failure. Amazingly, not many recipients appear to have died from complications.

Russia, 1682: the nobleman's skull

The first tissue xenograft was reputedly recorded in 1682 when a Russian nobleman, who had lost part of his scalp and skull in battle, had the loss "successfully repaired by a surgeon with a piece of bone taken from the skull of a dog." The Orthodox Church, however, believing that no man could be Christian if he had a dog bone in his head, threatened the nobleman with excommunication. A God-fearing man, he chose to have the fragments of the dog bone removed.

Over the centuries, a wide variety of animal tissues have been transplanted into human subjects. According to British surgeon Thomas Gibson, who himself carried out important work on skin grafting at the end of the Second World War, the list of animal tissues transplanted in ages past included tendons, bones, endocrine tissues such as the thyroid gland, and ovaries. A rabbit's eye was transplanted into a human on one occasion in 1887. And in 1896, a sheep's urethra was used in an attempt to repair a human urethra. Many more transplants involved skin, the extensive list of donors including dogs, cats, rabbits, rats, cockerels, chickens, pigeons, and most popular of all, frogs.

Chicago, 1880: Dr. Lee's lamb

Skin grafts were sometimes applied in the form of pedicled grafts—flaps of skin raised on the donor, one end of which was stitched to the recipient while the other end remained attached to the donor. When new blood vessels had grown into the skin flap from the recipient—which usually took a few weeks—the flap was completely detached from the donor. This technique is still used by plastic surgeons today; however, it is used only to move skin from one site to another on the same patient.

The enthusiasm for pedicled skin grafts was illustrated in 1860 by a British surgeon with a taste for animal experimentation. By creating raw areas on the back of a rat and the chest of a crow, he united the crow astride the back of the rat. Perhaps not surprisingly, he reported that "the crow scarcely possesses power of wing sufficient to raise its companion far from the ground, though it flutters along at the height of a foot or two for several yards." There have certainly been some strange experiments performed in the name of medicine or science!

In one incredible case reported from Chicago in 1880, three pedicled skin flaps from a living lamb were applied to the back of an extensively burned 10-year-old girl. The grafts were attached at one end to the little girl and at the other to the lamb. To prevent them from tearing apart, the lamb was "fastened in the standing posture, in a wood cage, its body being securely fixed and sustained by plaster of Paris bandaging of its limbs and quarters." The plan was to wait for new blood vessels from the little girl to grow into the skin flaps before cutting the flaps completely from the lamb. The child sadly died before the skin flaps were detached from the lamb. At autopsy, the flaps were optimistically said to be "fully adherent, and were capable of being nourished from the body of the child," clearly a flawed observation. (Six days after the operation was performed, and well before the little girl's death, the surgeon, Dr. E. W. Lee, submitted a report of the case to the *Boston Medical and Surgical Journal*. It seems that the desire for rapid publication among doctors was just as strong then as it is today—even when the outcome of their endeavors was not yet known.)

The late 1800s: the fashion for frogs

The use of free (unpedicled) skin grafts was much more popular than of pedicled grafts. Frogs were cheap and easily obtained. The skin had the advantage of not having hair, fur, or feathers and, although it was pigmented, doctors noted that a few days after transplantation the pigment disappeared. Gruesomely, the frog was not always killed before the skin was "donated." An assistant would sometimes hold the frog by the head and legs while the surgeon cut strips of skin from the hapless animal, the length of the strip being determined "by the steadiness with which the animal is held by the assistant."

The skin was used to cover raw areas, such as leg ulcers and burns, often with good effect. Indeed, a British Indian Army surgeon named Ranking performed such grafts on between 300 and 400 patients, "all with good results." His first effort was on himself—he claimed that it cured an "obstinate ulceration of the skin of the foot, which had resisted all treatment and [had hitherto] steadily refused to heal." Although it is inconceivable that any such grafts took permanently, it is quite likely that many of them were successful in allowing healing of the ulcer or burn over which they were applied. The temporary protection that the graft provided, and the extra care it received in the form of dressings and hygiene, may well have accelerated natural healing of the underlying raw area.

Much later, in the 1960s and 1970s, pig skin was used not infrequently in patients with extensive burns. By then, however, it was realized that the cover provided would be only temporary, but might protect the raw area until either the skin had regrown or a skin graft from elsewhere on the patient's body could be applied.

As illustrated by the above experiences, xenotransplantation, like all other aspects of medicine, has had a checkered past. Over the years there have been several "therapies" advocated in which animal cells of one sort or another are injected into humans. One well-known center is the Clinique La Prairie in Switzerland, which has specialized in the controversial area of "rejuvenation therapy" (in which Voronoff was a pioneer). Here various sheep cells, usually from a fetus, are administered by injection to individuals, many of whom claim to feel benefit, though their scientific effect and value have been hard to define.

Alexis Carrel and the Birth
of 20th-Century Transplantation o o o

It is not until the early part of the 20th century that we see reports of actual organ transplants (as opposed to tissue and skin) from animals to humans. All of these were doomed to early failure, but it is clear that a few men of great scientific vision foresaw the enormous benefits that xenotransplantation could bring. One such surgeon, the Frenchman Alexis Carrel (page 36), was the first to do significant experimental work in the field of transplantation (initially in Lyons and subsequently in Chicago and New York), and had an extremely perceptive view of what the future might hold. As early as 1902 he predicted "the replacement of a diseased organ by a healthy organ in order to treat, for example, Bright's disease [kidney failure] by replacing the diseased kidneys by healthy kidneys."

By 1907 his vision had extended to xenotransplantation; uncannily, he suggested a concept not very dissimilar to the use of the genetically engineered pigs that are being created today. After dismissing the use of apes as donors as being "impracticable," he went on to state, "The ideal method would be to transplant on man organs of animals easy to secure and operate on, such as hogs, for instance. But it would in all probability be necessary to immunize organs of the hog against the immune serum. The future of transplantation of organs for therapeutic purposes depends on the feasibility of hetero transplantation [xenotransplantation]."

Carrel's major claim to fame is that he developed techniques for joining together blood vessels, a surgical feat that had not been successful previously. It was this surgical triumph that opened the field for organ transplantation, and won him the Nobel Prize in Physiology and Medicine in 1912. He utilized his expertise in blood vessel surgery in a wide range of experimental efforts aimed at investigating organ transplantation.

(A little-known fact in relation to the work of Alexis Carrel is that Charles Lindbergh (seen with Carrel on page 36), who was the first person to fly solo across the Atlantic, developed an interest in the perfusion of organs with blood and other fluids and worked consistently with Carrel in his laboratory for a period of almost 30 years. His contributions formed some of the background to the development of the heart-lung machine used routinely today for open heart surgery.)

Carrel's innovative surgical techniques led others to sporadic attempts at organ xenotransplantation in human recipients in the first half of the 20th century, involving the use of a variety of donor species. During the last 40 years, a more scientific approach has been followed, and has involved kidney, heart, and liver xenotransplantation, as well as tissue and cellular transplants. As of the end of 1998, no fewer than 53 organ xenotransplants have been performed in human patients, of which 45 involved the use of nonhuman primate organs, with 8 organs taken from other mammalian species. Some of these attempts are reviewed below.

Transplantation of Animal Kidneys ○ ○ ○

Early attempts

The earliest attempt at transplantation of animal kidneys was probably in 1902 by Emerich Ullman in Vienna, who transplanted a pig kidney to blood vessels in the arm of a woman. Few details are known, although we do know that the kidney did not function. Three years later, a French surgeon named Princeteau inserted slices of rabbit kidney into the kidney of a child who was dying of renal failure. "The immediate results were excellent," he wrote, "the volume of urine increased; vomiting stopped . . . [but] on the sixteenth day the child died of pulmonary congestion." In retrospect, with the scientific information we have today, it is inconceivable that the kidney slices functioned at all; the child probably died of a massive accumulation of fluid in his body (related to the kidney failure).

Mathieu Jaboulay in 1906, also in France, attempted two kidney transplants using a pig and a goat as donor animals. The blood vessels from the kidney to the patient's arm were connected, but the kidney remained external to the skin. Neither kidney functioned. Jaboulay attributed his failures to the formation of clots in the blood vessels, which may have been related to the inadequate surgical technique used in the pre-Carrel era, although rapid rejection could have had the same result. Four years later, Ernst Unger not only transplanted a monkey kidney into a human but, quite remarkably, transplanted a stillborn baby's kidney into a baboon.

By the 1920s it had become obvious to even the most optimistic surgeon that a xenograft was doomed to early failure, and interest temporarily declined. In the late 1940s and early 1950s, attention turned towards the transplantation of human organs (allotransplantation), but soon a shortage of suitable donor organs was realized. This, one must remember, was in the era before brain death had become accepted as the standard for confirming the death of the potential donor, a development that did not take place until the late 1960s.

Louisiana, 1963: Keith Reemtsma and chimpanzee kidneys

It was during this period in the early 1960s, when donor organs were scarce and long-term dialysis using the artificial kidney machine had not been established, that Keith Reemtsma (page 36), at that time a professor of surgery at Tulane University in Louisiana, made the first truly scientific attempts at xenotransplantation. He performed 13 kidney transplants using chimpanzees as donors, transplanting both of the animal kidneys into the patient. The chimpanzees were obtained from military establishments, where they had been used in experiments relating to space flight, and also from circuses, where, because of advancing age or bad temper, they were no longer wanted. Most of the transplanted kidneys survived for periods of 9 to 60 days, with the patients dying primarily from infection, but one pair of kidneys functioned for almost nine months.

This one long-term survivor actually went back to work as a schoolteacher and led a fairly normal life until she died suddenly of what was believed to be an electrolyte imbalance in her body. It is likely that the chimpanzee kidneys did not function exactly as human kidneys and the electrolytes in her body became unbalanced, leading to cardiac arrest. An autopsy showed her transplanted kidneys to be virtually normal, with no features of rejection (Figure 3.3). This remarkable achievement is even more impressive when one considers how primitive were the immunosuppressive agents available to the transplant team at that time, which was long before the introduction of the efficient drugs available to us today. The best known of these, cyclosporine, was not used in patients until the very late 70s. Why

figure 3.3. *In the mid-1960s, chimpanzee kidneys were transplanted into 13 patients by surgeon Keith Reemtsma (see p. 36). One patient survived for nine months, and was able to return to work as a school-teacher, before succumbing from an uncertain cause, but possibly from an electrolyte imbalance. Remarkably, at necropsy, the transplanted chimpanzee kidneys (shown) showed no signs of rejection. (Courtesy of Keith Reemtsma, M.D.)*

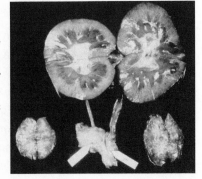

this one patient should have done so well in comparison with the others remains a mystery.

Colorado, 1964: Tom Starzl and baboon kidneys

Encouraged by Reemtsma's experience, transplant pioneer Thomas Starzl (page 36) and his colleagues in Denver used baboons as kidney donors. In general, the baboon kidneys were rejected slightly more vigorously than their chimpanzee counterparts, suggesting that the greater the evolutionary distance between donor and recipient, the more aggressive the rejection response. Six patients with baboon kidneys survived between 19 and 60 days, with the majority of deaths being from infection.

There were a few other isolated attempts during the 1960s. In several patients, the transplanted chimpanzee or baboon kidneys were noted to excrete very large amounts of urine during the first few days after transplantation. On some occasions, this was so great—up to 50 liters (13 gallons) in a 24-hour period—that it led to circulatory failure and death. There have been no attempts at kidney xenotransplantation within the past 30 years.

Transplantation of Animal Hearts o o o

The pioneering work of Christiaan Barnard (page 37), who performed the first human-to-human heart transplant in Cape Town in 1967, is well known. Less well known is the earlier effort by James Hardy (page 37) to transplant a chimpanzee heart into a human in 1964. Indeed, this was the first cardiac transplant of any type in a human subject.

Mississippi, 1964: James Hardy and the first chimpanzee heart transplant

A research group based at the University of Mississippi in Jackson had performed extensive experimental work on the technical aspects of heart transplantation (and had performed the world's first lung transplant in a human in the previous year, using a human donor lung). They chose a patient whose heart disease had progressed so far that he was on the point of death. They intended to use a human donor heart, but because the concept of brain death had not yet been accepted as a way of establishing which individuals were acceptable donors, no suitable human donor was available. Encouraged by

Reemtsma's recent experience with chimpanzee kidneys, they decided to go ahead with the transplant, using the heart from a chimpanzee.

The patient was a 68-year-old man who was in a semicomatose state. By today's criteria, he would certainly not be considered a suitable candidate for heart transplantation in view of his extremely poor general condition. But with no previous experience to guide them, it was not obvious to Hardy's surgical team that this almost certainly precluded a successful outcome. From a technical point of view, the transplant was successful, but the heart proved too small to support the patient's circulation. The chimpanzee weighed only 44 kg (96 lb), which was considerably less than the human recipient, and the heart could not pump enough blood to keep the man alive. Within two hours of the end of the operation, the patient was dead.

There was much media and medical criticism of Hardy's attempt, particularly with regard to the ethics of using animal organs. This criticism had considerable impact on Hardy's surgical team, and they did not carry out any further heart transplants.

London and Houston, 1968: pig and sheep heart grafts

Approximately six months after Christiaan Barnard's first attempt at human-to-human heart transplantation in 1967, two well-known heart surgeons in different parts of the world utilized animal hearts when no human heart was available. Denton Cooley in Houston, Texas, used a sheep heart, and Donald Ross, in London, England, used a pig heart to try to save the lives of patients who had unsuccessfully undergone open heart surgery and who would otherwise die upon being removed from the heart-lung machine. However, both transplanted animal hearts were rejected even before the operations were concluded. Another pig heart that Ross perfused with a a third patient's blood that same day, as a preliminary step before another transplant experiment was undertaken, ceased functioning almost immediately upon being exposed to the human blood.

The two surgeons gave surprisingly similar accounts of the appearance of the transplanted hearts, both of which were rejected within minutes. Cooley reported the sheep heart as going into "spasm," and Ross described the pig hearts as becoming absolutely "rigid." Those of us involved in experimental heart xenotransplantation have become accustomed to this ugly appearance. Rapid rejection causes rupture of blood vessels with bleeding into the heart muscle, giving the heart a black color and solid texture.

Donald Ross had the insight to use the pig heart he actually transplanted as an accessory heart in the hope that the patient's own heart would recover

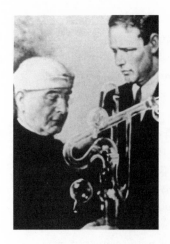

Alexis Carrel, Nobel Prize winner for medicine in 1912 for his work on the surgical joining of blood vessels, pictured with Charles Lindbergh, the well-known aviator (who was the first man to fly across the Atlantic Ocean), who assisted Carrel for many years in his experimental laboratory.

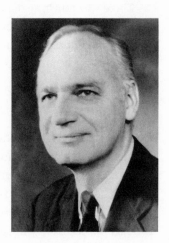

Keith Reemtsma, at that time a surgeon at Tulane University in Louisiana, was the first to attempt a series of chimpanzee kidney transplants in patients with end-stage renal failure. This was the first attempt at clinical xenotransplantation in modern times. (Courtesy of Keith Reemtsma, M.D.)

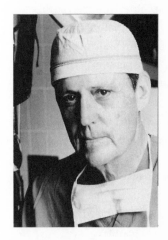

Tom Starzl, American liver transplant pioneer, attempted liver xenotransplantation in several patients using chimpanzee or baboon livers. In 1992, one patient with a transplanted baboon liver survived for 70 days. (Courtesy of Thomas Starzl, M.D.)

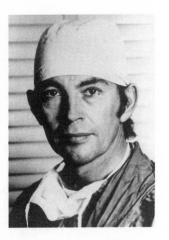

Christiaan Barnard, the University of Cape Town surgeon well known for establishing human-to-human heart transplantation in 1967, also carried out two auxiliary heart transplants using chimpanzee and baboon hearts, respectively, in 1977. (Photograph by Don MacKenzie.)

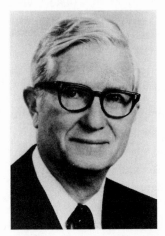

University of Mississippi surgeon James Hardy was the first to perform heart transplantation in a human patient (in 1964) when he utilized a chimpanzee heart. The heart failed and the patient died on the operating table. (Courtesy of James Hardy, M.D.)

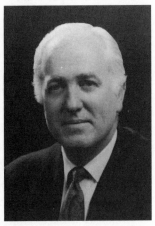

Leonard Bailey was the surgeon who performed the controversial baboon heart transplant in Baby Fae in 1984. (Courtesy of Leonard Bailey, M.D.)

within a few days, at which time the pig heart could be removed. This idea was a good one, but there was really no prospect that either of these animal hearts would survive for more than a few minutes or hours once perfused with human blood. To Donald Ross and his colleagues, however, must be credited the concept of using an animal heart as a "bridging" device towards transplantation with a human heart, an idea that was taken up subsequently by Barnard.

Both Cooley and Ross, eminent and distinguished surgeons, have mentioned to us that they are rather embarrassed by these premature attempts at xenotransplantation, which perhaps were spurred by the excitement and enthusiasm of that period, when heart transplantation was becoming more commonly (if generally unsuccessfully) performed at many centers throughout the world. In retrospect, they realize that evolution and biology were against them and failure was inevitable. But then every decision is easy with the aid of hindsight.

Cape Town, 1977: Christiaan Barnard's auxiliary hearts

Almost ten years later, in 1977, Barnard used chimpanzee and baboon hearts in the same way Ross had, as auxiliaries, in attempts to prolong the survival of patients who had just undergone unsuccessful open heart surgery, hoping that the patients' own hearts would recover. The chimpanzee heart functioned for four days but was then rejected; the patient died, as his own heart had not recovered. The baboon heart was not large enough to support the circulation satisfactorily, and the patient succumbed in the intensive care unit six hours later.

California, 1984: Leonard Bailey and Baby Fae

There was a gap of several years before the next attempt at cardiac xenotransplantation took place. During this period, the immunosuppressive drug cyclosporine had been introduced and had greatly improved the results of the transplantation of human organs. Encouraged by this fact, in 1984 a Loma Linda, California, group led by Leonard Bailey (page 37) used a baboon heart in a newborn baby known throughout the world as "Baby Fae" (Figure 3.4), who was born with a severely deformed heart. She survived for 20 days after the transplant, at which time the heart was rejected. The initial plan was to replace the xenografted heart with a human donor heart as soon as possible, using the xenograft only as a temporary support or bridging device, but no suitable human heart could be found before the child died.

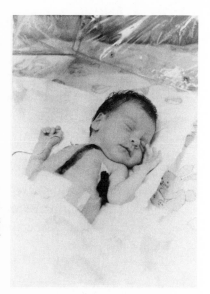

figure 3.4. *Baby Fae, born prematurely with a malformed heart, received a heart from a baboon in 1984. The operation was performed by Loma Linda University surgeon Leonard Bailey (see page 37). The heart was rejected and the baby died on the 20th post-transplant day. (Courtesy of Loma Linda University Medical Center, Loma Linda, California.)*

It is interesting to speculate whether the baboon heart might have survived longer had Baby Fae had a different blood type. The rules of organ transplantation are fundamentally identical to those governing blood transfusions: there must be blood group compatibility between donor and recipient. Baby Fae was of blood group O, and she would have needed a human donor heart from someone who also had type O blood. Baboon blood groups are confined to A, B, and AB, however, and so a baboon of blood type B had to be chosen as the donor for Baby Fae. This increased the chance of rejection of the heart and may well have played a role in the child's death. However, subsequent experimental research suggests that the immunosuppressive drugs available at that time may not have been powerful enough to prevent graft rejection even if the blood groups of donor and recipient had matched.

Poland, 1992, and India, 1996: the last attempts

There have been two recent attempts at heart xenotransplantation. In 1992 a pig heart was transplanted into a human in Sosnowiec, in Poland. The patient survived for almost 24 hours. Although this transplant was presumably carried out in a desperate life-saving attempt, with the state of knowledge as it was in 1992 there really was no realistic prospect that the patient would survive for any reasonable period of time.

The final effort was by a surgeon in northern India during late 1996. He also chose a pig heart for his patient, who died at the time of the operation.

Initially, there was doubt whether the transplant had actually taken place, but it seems that it did as the surgeon was jailed by the state authorities for allegedly flouting normal medical practice. Our last information (*The New Indian Express*, February 2, 1999) was that he was out of prison and had announced his intention to perform further xenotransplants.

Transplantation of Animal Livers o o o

The first documented attempt at liver xenotransplantation was by Tom Starzl and his colleagues in Denver in 1966. In the next eight years this group performed four chimpanzee liver transplants in humans, with the grafts surviving for up to 14 days. Other isolated unsuccessful attempts were documented during that period.

Pittsburgh, 1992: Tom Starzl and baboon livers

In 1992 and 1993 Starzl's team, by then based in Pittsburgh, again performed liver xenotransplantation, on these occasions using baboons as donors. The first of these two cases can be considered a relative success in that there was little evidence of rejection of the liver, which functioned for 70 days. But this was probably achieved at the expense of overly vigorous immunosuppression, as the patient died of overwhelming sepsis. The second case was less successful, as the patient never regained consciousness following the operation. Although there was again little evidence of rejection of the transplanted liver, the patient died after 27 days with a multitude of problems and failure of many of the body's vital organs.

These transplants were based on an interesting observation. Both patients were dying from liver failure caused by hepatitis B. When the failure is advanced, it is usually treated by transplantation using a human liver. However, the new transplanted human liver can also be attacked by the hepatitis B virus, which remains in the patient's body. This can lead to failure of the transplanted liver, and the patient is no better off than before the transplant. There is some evidence, however, that baboons' livers are resistant to infection by the hepatitis B virus. It was therefore hoped that if the baboon liver could be protected from rejection, damage caused by the hepatitis B virus would be avoided.

Unfortunately, neither patient lived long enough to prove this concept conclusively. In view of the disappointing results, further planned attempts were abandoned until more experimental research could be carried out.

Los Angeles, 1993: Leonard Makowka and a pig liver

There has been one subsequent attempt at liver xenotransplantation in a human patient. On this occasion, in 1993, the surgical team in Los Angeles, headed by Leonard Makowka, used a pig liver and placed it as an accessory to the patient's own liver, which was not removed, in the hope of keeping the young woman alive until a human donor could be found.

The patient was suffering from fulminant hepatic failure, which is very frequently fatal. In this disease, rapid and severe liver malfunction occurs, with the resultant accumulation in the body of harmful toxins that are the by-products of normal metabolism and which the liver usually renders harmless. The accumulation of these toxic metabolites leads to failure of brain function (encephalopathy), and the patient becomes comatose. In addition, essential amino acids and blood clotting factors are no longer manufactured by the diseased liver, resulting in rapid failure of the normal metabolism of the body, with spontaneous bleeding from the gastrointestinal tract, for example. Kidney failure usually follows, with an accumulation of fluid in the body. Swelling of the brain develops, increasing the pressure within the skull. Eventually, the brain is irreversibly compressed and death occurs.

Although the Los Angeles team's approach was an intelligent one, unfortunately the pig liver was rejected within a few hours and ceased to function. The patient's brain was injured by the accumulation of toxins that could not be cleared from her body by either her own liver or the pig liver, and she died before a human liver became available.

Maintaining Life by Animal Liver Perfusion o o o

Apart from the handful of animal livers that have actually been transplanted, there have been a much larger number of attempts (mainly in the United States and South Africa) to temporarily support a patient in liver failure by the use of animal livers that were not actually grafted into the patient's body. This has been attempted by a technique known as extracorporeal liver perfusion, in which the major blood vessels of the liver are connected to the patient's own blood vessels by flexible tubes. The patient's blood therefore circulates through the animal liver while it is outside the patient's body.

Although human livers have been used for such temporary support in the past, today these livers are reserved for transplantation. Animal livers have been and remain the preferred choice when only short-term liver support of this nature is required. The animal liver generally functions adequately for only a few hours, and then is rejected; a second animal liver is then used for a further period of time, either immediately or the next day. This can continue for several days, during which either a human donor liver becomes available, allowing transplantation, or the patient's own liver shows signs of recovery, which can occur in some cases of fulminant hepatic failure. These latter cases are usually those where the patient's liver has been seriously damaged by a chemical toxin absorbed from the gastrointestinal tract (such as by an overdose of certain prescription drugs) or by an overwhelming viral infection such as hepatitis. The liver, however, has great powers of recovery, and if the patient can be kept alive by a temporary liver, the patient may recover fully without any transplant.

The animal liver, be it from a pig, monkey, or baboon, has a better chance of resisting rapid rejection by the patient's immune system than might be anticipated. For a variety of reasons, the immune response, which is what causes rejection, is diminished in patients with liver failure. These patients' bodies are less able to mount an immune attack on the animal liver, which consequently functions for a longer period of time than would be expected.

In the 1960s and 1970s, several extracorporeal techniques were tried for the treatment of patients with fulminant hepatic failure, including cross-circulation, in which the patient's blood circulation was connected via tubes to that of a normal human or even to a nonhuman primate. This differed from extracorporeal liver perfusion in that the patient's blood passed through the entire body of the healthy "donor" (not just the liver), and the donor's blood in turn passed through the body of the patient. The normal liver of the healthy human or nonhuman primate would detoxify the blood of the patient. Experience soon demonstrated, however, that neither cross-circulation nor any of the other techniques were any more effective in reversing the deep encephalopathy that occurred in these patients than extracorporeal perfusion using an animal liver.

Significant, if limited, experience with extracorporeal liver perfusion has shown us that livers from various animal species can reverse deep coma in a patient with fulminant hepatic failure. First, at least temporary recovery of consciousness occurs in approximately one-third of patients, and improvement in the level of consciousness in a further 10 to 15%. Second, perfusion using a pig liver is less successful than that with a baboon liver. This can be illustrated by the fact that a baboon liver can provide support for up to approximately 24 hours, whereas a pig liver generally functions satisfactorily for only 5 to 12 hours. This difference is almost certainly related to the more rapid rejection of the pig liver. Third, when recovery from coma is achieved, it is sustained longer after baboon liver perfusion than after pig liver perfusion.

One of the pioneers in this field of therapy, transplant surgeon George Abouna, advocates this technique as a logical and cost-effective method of supporting a patient with fulminant hepatic failure in the hope that his or her own liver will recover. It allows human donor livers to be allocated to patients whose liver failure is irreversible. With the possibility of using livers from pigs that have been transgenically modified to resist rapid rejection, as discussed in Chapter 7, interest in this technique is being reborn.

Looking Back o o o

The results of clinical organ xenotransplantation have been disappointing. With the one exception of Keith Reemtsma's patient who lived for almost nine months supported by a pair of chimpanzee kidneys, no patient who received a whole-organ xenotransplant has lived longer than 70 days. When an organ has been used from any animal species other than a nonhuman primate, the results have been exceedingly poor, with no patient surviving even for one day. And although patients have survived the xenotransplantation of tissues or cells, there has in general been little evidence of long-term survival or function of the transplanted animal cells. The exceptions have mostly been cases in which animal cells were injected into the brains of human patients with degenerative brain disease.

Given our record to date, at first glance it would certainly take an optimist to believe that we can overcome the problems we face. In the remainder of this book, however, we shall explore the several ways in which scientists, physicians, and surgeons are currently attempting to overcome these barriers, and the reasons many of those conducting research in this field are cautiously optimistic that the problems will be solved within the near future. Indeed, significant progress has already been made.

chapter 4

All Animals Are Equal, but Some Are More Equal than Others

The choice of donor

No Longer Science Fiction o o o

The large building is made up of a number of rooms, each divided into pens by concrete walls that rise to waist or shoulder height. When not wandering about on the stone floors, the pigs are generally eating and drinking from the food and water containers fixed along the walls. There are about 50 pigs altogether, and they look and sound like any other pigs with always a few grunting and squealing. But if we could look inside them, we would see something very strange, indeed: *human* proteins on the surface of the cells that line the blood vessels throughout their entire body, in all of their organs. These are "humanized" pigs—until recently a science fiction dream, but now firmly part of real-life science and medicine.

The pig is considered by many surgeons as the most likely answer to the donor organ shortage—maybe not necessarily "humanized" pigs, although it is likely they will play a major role. Why the pig? Wouldn't chimpanzees or baboons be preferable? After all, they are the closest relatives of man, much closer on the evolutionary tree than the pig, and, as we have seen, experimental data show that using organs from animals genetically more similar to us reduces the problem of rejection.

Let us consider our choices. What criteria should we seek in the ideal organ donor for humans?

Candidate Number 1: The Great Apes o o o

The closeness of the phylogenetic relationships between the great apes and humans is illustrated by the fact that their DNA sequences, the genetic blueprint of all life, differ from ours by only about 2%. This is the reason for the far greater compatibility between human and nonhuman primate tissues than between humans and other mammals, such as the pig. If it were purely the immune response that was the deciding factor, then we would clearly choose one of the great apes, such as the chimpanzee. However, this is only one of many factors that have to be considered in selecting a potential donor animal. (Strictly speaking, the animals that will provide the organs for transplantation are not "donors," as donation is a voluntary act. "Source animals" is a preferable term. Nevertheless, in this book, the two terms will be used interchangeably.)

The great apes, such as the gorilla, chimpanzee, orangutan, and even the gibbon, are now endangered species and are clearly not available in the numbers necessary to fulfill the requirements of organ transplantation worldwide. Although we could breed them in captivity, such a plan would prove exceedingly time-consuming and immensely expensive, as we shall see when we consider the baboon as a source of organs.

Even if the great apes were available in the necessary numbers, because of their physical and behavioral similarity to humans many people oppose their use as sources of organs for transplantation. This would almost certainly jeopardize any xenotransplantation program that was initiated. But the whole issue of the rights and wrongs of the use of great apes as sources of organs for humans is mooted at present by their scarcity. Despite their very close relationship with humans, which would make therapeutic measures to overcome rejection much easier—as Keith Reemtsma discovered in the 1960s—we clearly have to rule them out as potential organ donors.

Candidate Number 2: The Baboon o o o

In view of the small numbers of great apes let us move down the evolutionary tree to consider the larger Old World monkeys. The baboon is a nonhuman primate that still survives in sufficient numbers in the wild to be considered as a potential donor of organs for humans. But microbiologists—experts in bacteria and viruses—are, to put it far too mildly, hesitant to allow us to use wild-caught baboons or monkeys as donors of organs for humans. Jonathan Allen, of the Southwest Foundation for Biomedical Research in Texas, is one of those who are fearful that baboon viruses might cause serious infection in humans, which could conceivably spread to AIDS-like proportions. (Indeed, HIV is now thought to have originated in nonhuman primates; see below.)

Baboons living in the wild are in an uncontrolled microbiological environment and susceptible to infection with bacteria and viruses from the other animal species, including insects, rodents, and birds, with whom they share their habitat. For example, the gibbon ape lives high in the forest in Southeast Asia and is generally not in contact with rodents on the forest floor. However, a retrovirus that was somehow transferred from the rodents resulted in a leukemia-like condition in infected apes.

Allen's forceful publicizing of the risks he and others see if baboon organs are placed into human bodies has at times won him no friends among the transplant surgeons aggressively pursuing xenotransplantation. These surgeons had become increasingly frustrated and distressed by watching the patients on their transplant waiting lists decline and die for want of human donor organs. But slowly Allen's message has been accepted by the majority (though not all) of these surgeons, who have come to accept, if sometimes reluctantly, his expert opinion of the risks such transplants hold. Whether his fears are justified or not we shall probably now never know, but he deserves every credit for vociferously raising his concerns at a time when one or two groups were on the brink of transplanting more baboon organs into human patients.

The risk of the spread of baboon viruses is thought to be much higher if wild baboons are used than if they are bred and reared in captivity under conditions where they can be monitored closely. Baboons could conceivably be bred in closed colonies in sufficient numbers to provide for our projected needs. This would certainly be easier and cheaper than breeding chimpanzees in equivalent numbers. There are already several primate breeding establishments in the United States, including one in Texas with over 2,500 monkeys and baboons in residence. The baboon, however, does not fulfill many of our requirements (Table 4.1).

Disadvantages

The first mark against the baboon is size. Even the largest of adult male baboons is rarely more than 40 kg (88 lb) in weight, and some of their organs, such as the heart and lungs, would not be large enough to adequately support the life of a large adult human, who may weigh in excess of 80 to 100 kg (176 to 220 lb). A pair of kidneys from a large baboon, however, would probably be sufficient to support a full-grown human. The liver has great powers of regeneration, as demonstrated by the two baboon liver transplants per-

table 4.1

Relative Advantages and Disadvantages of Baboons and Pigs as Potential Donors of Organs and Tissues for Humans

	Baboon	*Pig*
Availability	Limited	Unlimited
Breeding potential	Poor	Good
Period to reproductive maturity	3–5 years	4–8 months
Length of pregnancy	173–193 days	114 ± 2 days
Number of offspring	1–2	5–12
Growth	Slow (9 years to reach maximum size)	Rapid (adult human size within 6 months)**
Size of adult organs	Inadequate*	Adequate
Cost of maintenance	High	Significantly lower
Anatomical similarity to humans	Close	Moderately close
Physiological similarity to humans	Close	Moderately close
Relationship of immune system to humans	Close	Distant
Knowledge of tissue typing	Limited	Considerable (in selected herds)
Necessity for blood type compatibility with humans	Important	Probably unimportant
Experience with genetic engineering	None	Considerable
Risk of transfer of infection (xenozoonosis)	High	Low
Availability of specific pathogen-free animals	No	Yes
Public opinion	Mixed	More in favor

*The size of certain organs, e.g., the heart, would be inadequate for transplantation into adult humans.
**Breeds of miniature swine are approximately 50% of the weight of domestic pigs at birth and sexual maturity, and reach a maximum weight of approximately 30% of standard breeds.

formed by Tom Starzl and his group in Pittsburgh, and will grow in size rapidly over the course of a few weeks. A baboon liver would therefore probably provide sufficient function to support the life of an adult human.

Secondly, most baboon pregnancies end in only one offspring, occasionally two, and therefore breeding programs would have to be very extensive to provide 50,000 or more organs a year, as may well be necessary. Very large numbers of baboons bred in captivity would be required to supply these needs. Furthermore, baboons do not reach sexual maturity before three to five years of age, and the length of the average pregnancy of a baboon is approximately six months, making the creation of large colonies very time-consuming. The baboon also takes approximately nine years to grow to full adult size; it would be extremely expensive to maintain large numbers of animals until they reached a sufficient size to be used for transplantation purposes, and this would mean that baboon organs would be exceedingly expensive.

In their favor, baboon organs are similar to human organs both anatomically and physiologically and in general would be expected to function very adequately if transplanted into humans. There are, however, certain problematic differences. For example, Starzl's group noted that the bile produced by the baboon livers transplanted into humans was very thick. This is not related to the natural consistency of baboon bile, as baboon bile is similar to human bile when analyzed chemically, but the changes in consistency are almost certainly related to its production in a foreign environment, namely, a human body, which in some way alters the nature of the baboon bile. Such potential incompatibilities between animal species and humans are discussed further in Chapter 10.

The risk of infection

Even with colony-bred baboons, the risk of infection remains a major concern. As nonhuman primates have been kept in captivity for relatively short periods of time when compared with domesticated farm animals, viruses picked up in the wild may well persist, even through many generations of captivity.

Let us consider this in more detail. There is a growing awareness that some of the serious viruses that afflict humans have their origin in nonhuman primates in the wild. The best example is the human immunodeficiency viruses, which cause AIDS and which are believed to have arisen in nonhuman primate species in Africa and in some way were transferred to humans. There are other examples of nonhuman primate viruses—so-called simian viruses—that intermittently cause fatal infections in the human population; the herpes B virus is one such example.

The potential for simian viral epidemics in the human community is such that we would have to take steps to ensure that any baboon donors absolutely did not carry any such known viruses. Of even more concern to Jonathan Allen and other leading virologists, however, is that there may be other dangerous simian viruses of which we remain ignorant and for which there are currently no diagnostic tests. What worries some experts even more than the possibility that the human recipient of the organ might develop a life-threatening infection is the possibility that the recipient may transfer the virus to those around him before his own infection becomes clinically apparent. The outcome could be a catastrophe of enormous proportions.

There are those who suggest that the risk of transmitting hitherto unknown but lethal viruses from apes to humans is small or even negligible, but it must be remembered that not very many years ago we were unaware of the existence of the AIDS viruses. Although we shall never be able to limit every single such risk, we clearly have to heed the warnings of experts in this field. (This topic is discussed in more detail in Chapter 11.)

Public opinion

As we've seen, some of the disadvantages of harvesting organs from baboons—indeed, all nonhuman primates—are purely logistic and some are related to the potential risks involved. Additionally, the public reaction to the use of baboons as organ donors has to be considered. Although baboons are a little further removed phylogenetically from humans than are chimpanzees, they still have many human characteristics. A significant and vociferous segment of the public would oppose the planned killing of large numbers of baboons even if their organs would be life-saving to dying humans. As with the great apes, public opinion must be very carefully considered; if adverse, it would prevent, delay, or greatly complicate the establishment of organ xenotransplantation.

Candidate Number 3: The Pig ○ ○ ○

The risk of controversy with regard to the use of animals as organ donors for humans would be minimized if the animal chosen was already being killed in large numbers on a daily basis to provide food for human consumption.

Animals of adequate but not excessive size in this group would include the pig and the sheep. Pigs have several advantages over sheep, such as the ease with which a large number can be bred and housed under clean conditions.

The immunological barriers presented by the use of pig organs are significantly greater, however, than those provided by the baboon. The major problem is the presence in the human of antibodies directed against pig tissues (anti-pig antibodies), which initiate the rapid rejection of the pig organ. This phenomenon is rare when a baboon organ is transplanted, as humans do not have high levels of anti-baboon antibodies in their blood. If, for the purposes of the present discussion, we exclude this immunological disadvantage, the pig can be seen to have many advantages over the baboon (Table 4.1).

Advantages

As pigs are already slaughtered in very large numbers to provide food for humans (almost 100 million annually in the United States alone) and have been so for centuries, there would be substantially less public controversy with regard to the use of pigs as organ donors. (The ethics of the use of animal donors is discussed further in Chapter 13.)

Pigs produce litters of 5 to 10, or more, at a time, and the animals reach reproductive maturity within six months. Sows are ready to mate every three weeks, which is a major advantage when developing a strain with special characteristics, which might include modifications induced by genetic engineering. Pregnancy lasts less than four months (three months, three weeks, and three days, to be exact), making the buildup of a suitable herd relatively rapid. Pigs are easy and cheap to maintain, and rapidly grow to a size that would be sufficient to provide organs for the largest of adult humans. Within six months of birth, pigs are as big as a fully grown human, and by one year they are even larger. Various breeds of miniature swine (sometimes called pigmees!) that at maturity weigh about as much as a large adult human (100–130 kg or 220–260 lb) are available. All of these factors would greatly reduce the cost of providing organs from pigs when compared to baboons.

Despite the phylogenetic distance between humans and swine, pig anatomy and physiology are surprisingly similar to those of humans. For example, both pigs and humans are omnivorous—that is, they eat a meat and vegetable diet—and both have a propensity to obesity. Pigs have been used as research animals, and their physiology has been extensively studied, particularly with regard to the cardiovascular system. (This is not to say that there are not some significant physiological or metabolic differences that may provide major hurdles, as we shall discuss in Chapter 10.) Some observers have even pointed out certain similarities between the eating habits and social behavior of the two species!

Potential for genetic engineering

Certain of the advantages of the pig compared to the baboon—shorter pregnancy, larger litters, shorter period for sows to reach reproductive maturity—augur well for our ability to genetically engineer the donor animal to reduce the possibility of rejection. Here we return to the "humanized" pig. Scientists are increasingly looking at ways whereby the donor animal can be modified by transgenic techniques to minimize attack by the human recipient's immune system; such endeavors are discussed later in this book. It should also be noted that if techniques such as cloning prove fully successful, then the situation may change dramatically, and it may become possible to produce greatly modified baboons as rapidly as modified pigs.

The risk of infection

One might presume that because humans have lived close to pigs for centuries, farming and slaughtering them, and have eaten pigs in huge numbers, that there are few bacteria and viruses that the pig carries that are readily transferable to humans. It should not be forgotten, however, that the influenza pandemic that swept through the world in 1918 and killed between 20 million and 40 million people was possibly an influenza virus that commonly infects only pigs, not humans. Experts insist, however, that the fact that humans are relatively rarely infected with swine microorganisms does not preclude the possibility of transfer of an infectious agent when an organ is transplanted from the pig directly into a human body. From a microbiological standpoint, this is a very different situation from external contact between human and pig.

For centuries, infections have been passed from farm animals to humans, usually by direct contact. Examples include brucellosis (from the cow) and anthrax (from sheep). To differentiate these from infections that are transferred exclusively between humans, these animal-to-human infections have been termed "zoonoses." Similarly, animals can be infected by direct contact with humans; it is well known, for example, that handlers of animals, including baboons and pigs, can transfer tuberculosis to them. Such an infection can rapidly be lethal to the infected animal, which has no immune defense to this new infection. Indeed, such an infection can rapidly spread throughout an entire colony of baboons or herd of pigs.

If xenotransplantation becomes scientifically feasible, there will be a possibility of transferring infection with the transplanted organ. The warm, nourishing human body may provide ideal conditions for growth of some swine microorganisms. Furthermore, the transferred microorganisms are likely to come into direct contact with the blood, which may transport them effortlessly to all parts of the host's body. The infection may therefore not be confined to the transplanted organ. To differentiate this type of infection from the usual zoonosis, the terms "xenozoonosis" or "xenosis" have been suggested.

Pigs have been reared under relatively controlled conditions for generations, and in recent years herds free of specific pathogens, such as tuberculosis, have been established. Nevertheless, the pig can harbor bacteria, viruses, fungi, and parasites that can cause disease and undoubtedly could lead to infection in humans if transferred with the transplanted organ. In general, however, microbiologists are significantly less worried about the potential of an AIDS-like epidemic following the transplantation of pig organs than baboon organs.

Pig diseases and defects

Infectious diseases in swine are only one concern, albeit a major one. We also need to consider other potential complications from the use of the pig as an organ donor. Are there disease processes that affect its organs that might lead to dysfunction of the organ after transplantation into a human? Like any species, pigs suffer from certain diseases and disorders. For example, they can be born with heart defects, though the incidence is very low. As there is a genetic foundation for many such birth defects, it should be possible to reduce this low incidence even further by selective breeding. Are pig cancers common, and might there be a risk of transfer of cancerous cells with the organ to the human recipient? Fortunately, the incidence of cancer in swine is very low (occurring in only approximately 0.004%, or 4 in every 100,000, of the pigs in the United States). As the incidence of cancer increases as a population ages, cancer would become more common if pigs were allowed to survive into middle life, which, as the dinner table awaits them, they generally are not. For transplantation, we will be using the organs from young pigs within the first year or two of life, and therefore the risk of transfer of a cancerous tumor should be extremely low.

Tissue typing in pigs

Certain herds of pigs have one other great advantage—our knowledge of their tissue typing—that could not be matched in baboons for generations unless cloning becomes commonplace. At least two such herds in the United States have been studied in great detail.

A human can be tissue-typed by a simple test using white blood cells, which have on their surface molecules—known as antigens—that give the individual his or her specific tissue type. There is considerable variation in antigens between one human and another, and the closeness of the tissue match between prospective donor and recipient predicts, to a considerable extent, how long an organ transplanted from one to the other is likely to survive.

Pigs can also be typed in a similar way, and we have considerable information about their tissue types, more than any other suitable large animal. Although we are not yet at a stage where we can make full use of this information, it is likely to prove invaluable in the future success of xenotransplantation.

By far the most extensive study of the relationship of tissue type to organ transplantation in the pig has been by immunologist David Sachs and his colleagues, formerly at the National Institutes of Health in Bethesda, Maryland, and now at Massachusetts General Hospital in Boston. When organ transplantation is performed between pigs (i.e., pig allografting), matching for certain tissue antigens results in a much reduced rejection response than when there is no such matching. For example, human and pig tissue antigens can both be divided into Class I and Class II types. In pigs, if there is compatibility between donor and recipient Class II antigens, then organ allografts exchanged between these pigs have a very high chance of excellent long-term survival, irrespective of how well the Class I antigens match up.

It is possible that certain pig tissue types may prove more compatible as donors for humans than other types—that is, those tissue types may be rejected by humans less vigorously than others. If this were found to be the case, we would clearly have to select and breed pigs of this type. Although this concept is not yet proven, it would seem wise to begin by concentrating our attention on these few herds where inbreeding has resulted in very close similarity, approaching identity, between the tissue types of individual pigs and in which the tissue type is well documented. Perhaps surprisingly, not all groups involved in xenotransplantation research are doing so, even though these strains of pig have been offered to all who might wish to use them.

A related issue is ABO blood group compatibility, which is of great importance in blood transfusion and organ transplantation between humans or when a nonhuman primate donor is used for a human recipient. This is much less important if a pig is the donor, as the pig's blood group antigen expression appears relatively weak. Nevertheless, herds have been bred in which all of the pigs are of blood group O, the universal donor blood type. As O-type blood and organs are acceptable to *all* human recipients, there will be no risk of rejection of the organ by the human recipient on the basis of ABO incompatibility, no matter what the blood type of the human patient.

Pig upward mobility

In the last 10 years there has been a quantum leap in the status of pigs in the eyes of many. No longer the lowly farmyard hog wallowing in mud and eating slop discarded from the human table, and considered by some groups to be too unclean to be eaten, the pig has become the center of a growing scientific and biotechnological endeavor. Its status has been elevated to that of a research source of the highest order. And plans are afoot to raise its status even higher by further sophisticated inbreeding, by genetic engineering and cloning to "humanize" it, and by ultimately rendering it disease-free. It will be housed in conditions second to none in the animal kingdom. Its every whim will be catered to. And if xenotransplantation proves ultimately successful, the expression "pearls before swine" may come to be used not as a way of characterizing wastefulness but as an expression of thanksgiving.

chapter 5

Zero Tolerance

The rejection of animal organs

The Power of Nature ○ ○ ○

The surgeon completes the transplant of the pig heart into the baboon, just as surgeons Donald Ross and Denton Cooley did back in 1968, when they inserted pig and sheep hearts, respectively, into their human patients. The pig heart initially becomes a healthy pink color as the recipient's blood flows through it. It begins to beat. But, after as little as two minutes, the surgeon watches as it becomes a mottled, dusky blue color, and the contractions become weak and irregular. Blood ceases to flow through the organ as the small capillaries in the heart muscle become occluded by clots. The blood vessels rupture, and the heart rapidly swells due to the leakage of blood and fluid into the muscle wall. The heart stops beating. It is now an ugly black mass.

The surgeon has witnessed the most powerful immunological reaction that the human body can mount, a response initially developed millions of years ago in primitive animal species as a defense against invading microorganisms, largely bacteria and viruses. This innate immunological response has become a reflex reaction to the foreign threat, requiring little or none of the sophistication of the other human immunological response, the "cognate" or "adaptive" response, which, in evolutionary terms, has developed much more recently. The cognate response, which is involved in the rejection of transplanted human organs, requires the complex involvement of specialized cells that are present in mammals but not in primitive animal species. (Pig heart valves that are surgically placed in patients with defective valves do not undergo this rapid destruction because they consist largely of dead cells that have been processed to preserve them.)

For many years, researchers in this field felt completely helpless when faced by the body's powers to rapidly destroy what it perceives as being foreign and potentially harmful. We frequently speak of the "power of nature," but are usually referring to the strength of a hurricane or the violence of a tornado. But nature also reveals its power every day of our lives within our bodies, as our immune system constantly protects us against invading microorganisms. The overwhelming force of the immune system and its almost immediate and total destruction of an unwanted foreign organ is a perfect example of nature's fury when aroused.

It is this fury that has to be tamed if we are to achieve our goal of solving the shortage of donor organs by the use of animals such as the pig. We must learn to prevent the innate immune response that has been part of our natural mammalian defenses for millennia. In the words of the German scientist Claus Hammer, we have to learn how to "outwit evolution." This task is unlike much of medicine, where we are frequently fighting to correct a state in which our natural defense mechanisms have failed, to excise a cancerous growth from the stomach, for example. If we are to achieve xenotransplantation, we must overcome one of the human body's oldest and strongest natural survival mechanisms. It should come as no surprise, therefore, that our previous attempts at xenotransplantation were so dismally unsuccessful.

Let us first review briefly what happens when a human organ is transplanted into another human (allotransplantation). Rejection of the organ is much slower than the almost immediate destruction of an animal organ. Allograft rejection involves the more sophisticated cognate immune response—a response that has been relentlessly honed and refined over millions of years and is today a complex biological machine. As we learn more about this mechanism of rejection, an immunological puzzle of increasing complexity and sophistication is gradually emerging. It would take another book to describe the myriad of cells and molecules involved in the process of rejection. For this reason, only the bare essentials of the rejection process will be outlined here.

Rejection of Human Organs ○ ○ ○

When a patient receives a human organ, two potential rejection hurdles have to be overcome: an *acute* reaction, which occurs relatively rapidly over a few days or weeks, and a *chronic* reaction, which develops over months or years.

The term *hyperacute*, which we shall use later, refers to a process that is extremely rapid, occurring within minutes or hours. The violent rejection of an animal organ is one such hyperacute response.

The first hurdle: acute rejection

A newly transplanted organ is recognized by the recipient (also called the host) as being foreign—or what has been termed "non-self," as opposed to "self." But the body cannot differentiate between a foreign human organ and foreign microorganisms that might cause infection. Therefore, the body takes steps to destroy the transplanted tissue. As the host has generally not been exposed to a foreign organ previously, the sophisticated cognate mechanism of rejection is brought into play to destroy the intruder. Unless the recipient has been primed, or sensitized, to another human organ previously, he or she has to build up an attack over several days. This immune response is carried out mainly by a group of white blood cells known as T lymphocytes. They travel in the blood to the grafted organ, which they invade and destroy. This response is therefore variously termed "cellular rejection" (as cells are involved), "acute rejection" (as it develops relatively rapidly over only a few days), or, to give it its full title, "acute cellular rejection." Hereafter, these terms will be used interchangeably.

If no drugs are used to dampen the recipient's immune system, it takes only about a week for a transplanted human organ to be totally destroyed. During this period, its function will steadily deteriorate until it ceases to work altogether. If it is a life-supporting organ such as the heart, the patient will, of course, die. We have few data on this phenomenon in human subjects because patients are always treated with immunosuppressive drugs to prevent rejection. But in experimental animals, such as the mouse, rat, dog, or baboon, we have considerable evidence as to the mechanism by which this rejection is brought about.

Most of the immunosuppressive drugs we utilize in clinical transplantation (that is, in patients) are geared to suppressing the response of these T lymphocytes. If we administer a drug that destroys or inhibits the patient's T cells, they will obviously be prevented from destroying the transplanted organ.

Tissue typing in humans

The major molecules in the donor organ that are recognized by the body as foreign, and which activate the response by the recipient's T cells, are proteins that are commonly called antigens. Tissue typing, by which one individual's antigens can be differentiated from those of another individual, is performed by identifying them on the person's white blood cells.

Tissue typing nowadays is so accurate that it is being used on a daily basis to determine the parentage of children where there is doubt or legal controversy over the identity of the father (or, much more rarely, of the mother, particularly in cases where in vitro fertilization has occurred). In the case of a paternity determination, the child's tissue type is compared with that of the presumed father and known mother. On the basis of the results, the odds of the child being the progeny of that particular man can be determined with a high degree of accuracy, particularly if this information is taken into consideration with other factors, such as the ABO blood types of parents and child.

Before an organ transplant is performed, the ABO blood type and the tissue type of both the recipient and donor are determined. With very few exceptions, it is essential that the ABO types of the donor and patient be compatible, or rejection can occur rapidly. With regard to the tissue type, the rules are not so rigid. Whenever possible, an effort is made by the transplant team to match the recipient with a donor of similar tissue type. If the types are identical, as when an organ is transplanted between identical twins, the host T cells recognize the transplanted organ as "self" and take no steps to reject or destroy it. The greater the disparity between recipient and donor, the stronger is the rejection response.

Unfortunately, tissue typing takes several hours to perform. Although it is always possible to type the recipient while he or she is awaiting a transplant, it is sometimes not possible to type the donor before the actual transplant operation takes place. A brain-dead human donor is frequently in an unstable hemodynamic state—that is, the heart may be failing despite increasing support with drugs. If the organs are to be excised and transplanted before the heart fails completely, there may be insufficient time for donor tissue typing. If the heart stops beating, blood and oxygen will no longer be pumped to the other organs, which will suffer damage and no longer be suitable for transplantation. Indeed, time constraints may not allow donor typing with organs such as the heart, lungs, and liver, which all have to be transplanted as soon as possible. With kidneys, which can be safely stored in ice for 24 to 48 hours after removal, tissue typing and matching is performed in almost every case. If we could develop better methods of storing hearts, lungs, and livers, then matching of the recipient with the donor could always be carried out. This would almost certainly lead to longer survival of these grafted organs.

The second hurdle: chronic rejection

Chronic rejection is generally a slow, insidious process, frequently developing over a period of many months or years. For example, the host's response causes thickening of the walls of the arteries within the organ. Eventually the process leads to complete obstruction of the blood flow, which in turn results in the death of cells within the graft—for example, of the muscle cells of a transplanted heart. When enough cells have been killed, the graft eventually fails to function satisfactorily. The changes need not be limited to the blood vessels; chronic rejection can affect, for example, the airways in the lung, and various structures in the kidney and liver.

The exact cause(s) of chronic rejection and the mechanism by which it develops remain uncertain and controversial. It may be mediated by a combination of the effects of both cells (such as T lymphocytes) and antibodies on the transplanted organ. However, there is some evidence that factors other than rejection, such as viral infection, may also play a role.

Despite lifelong immunosuppressive drug therapy, most patients eventually develop chronic rejection of the grafted organ. It is the major cause of late graft failure. For example, about half of patients lose their heart or kidney graft function within 10 years of the transplant. When chronic rejection is advanced, retransplantation with a new organ is the only treatment that will keep the patient alive—unless, of course, it is a transplanted kidney that is undergoing rejection, in which case the patient can stay alive by using a dialysis machine to filter waste products from the blood.

Rejection in a "sensitized" recipient

The above descriptions of rejection relate to the course of events that take place in the vast majority of patients who receive an organ allograft. However, there is another form of rejection that we should consider, even though it occurs in only a handful of patients (much less than 1%). This is an ultrarapid or hyperacute form of rejection that is of great interest, as it is very similar, if not identical, to the violent rejection that takes place when a pig or sheep organ is transplanted into a human.

In these cases, rejection within minutes or hours is associated with an attack on the transplanted organ by antibodies rather than T cells. The first potential cause is when the organ recipient and donor are of incompatible ABO blood types. The organ can then be rejected by antibodies against the incompatible A or B antigens, which are sugars on the surface of the lining of the blood vessels of the grafted organ. A second cause is when the recipient has preexisting antibodies that react against the tissue type of the donor. These antibodies may have developed after a previous organ transplant, although such sensitization is by no means inevitable. But they can also develop in a pregnant woman who becomes sensitized to the antigens of the father that are present in the fetus she is carrying. Furthermore, patients who receive blood transfusions may develop antibodies against the tissue antigens on the foreign white cells in the blood.

If a subsequently transplanted organ shares some of the same antigens against which the patient has become sensitized, the second organ can be rejected extremely rapidly. In order to anticipate whether this is likely to happen, tests are carried out when a person's name is placed on the waiting list. If any antibodies against foreign human tissues are detected, when an organ donor becomes available it is essential to know the blood group and tissue type of the donor. Even better is to carry out an emergency test in which the serum of the potential recipient's blood is tested specifically against the donor white blood cells. If the donor cells are destroyed by the recipient serum, then generally the transplant is abandoned and the organ is offered to another patient who does not have antibodies against the donor cells. Since this is now standard practice, the incidence of hyperacute rejection of a transplanted human organ is extremely low.

Rejection of Animal Organs ○ ○ ○

The body's response to a transplanted animal organ depends largely on whether the organ is from an animal closely related to us, for example, a monkey or chimpanzee, or from a very disparate species such as the pig or sheep. In either case, the pattern of rejection is even more complex than when a human organ has been transplanted. The description that follows has therefore been greatly simplified.

Regardless of the donor species, acute cellular rejection is likely to occur, as in an allograft, and we believe that chronic rejection will also subsequently develop. However, in addition, early rejection due to the presence of antibodies also occurs in some form or other *in every case*. The nature of this early antibody-mediated response depends on the nature of the donor animal. If the donor organ is from a distantly related animal, such as the pig, a very rapid or hyperacute destruction occurs, as described at the beginning of this chapter. If the baboon or another primate closely related to humans is the donor, hyperacute rejection is generally not seen, although a slightly delayed response develops within two or three days. If these early forms of rejection can be avoided or treated, cellular rejection is seen later, as in human-to-human organ transplants.

Before examining the response to a xenotransplanted organ in more detail, let us comment briefly on antibodies. Antibodies are manufactured by the counterpart of the T lymphocytes, the B lymphocytes, which mature into particularly productive plasma cells. It has been estimated that a healthy body produces approximately 150 billion B lymphocytes each day, and that each B cell/plasma cell is capable of producing 2,000 antibody molecules every second! Humans, and indeed other mammals, have the ability to manufacture antibodies against any invading organism (for example, bacteria) or foreign protein (such as with a transplanted organ) introduced into their bodies. Antibodies produced against invading bacteria or viruses are, of course, beneficial to us. Unfortunately, antibodies produced against a transplanted organ are not.

Transplantation between closely related animals

Humans have no or very low levels of antibodies directed against other primates, such as chimpanzees or baboons, but after exposure to transplanted tissues, antibodies are produced rapidly. Without treatment, therefore, a nonhuman primate organ transplanted into a human would generally be destroyed by antibodies or by a combined antibody-cellular attack within days. The immunosuppressive drugs that we have available at present have some effect in delaying this form of rejection, although they are not as effective as they are against acute cellular rejection. Newer drugs currently in various stages of development may be more effective.

There is, therefore, a likelihood that an organ transplanted from a closely related species, such as a baboon, would function in a human for at least some months if the right combination of immunosuppressive drugs is administered. However, large doses of these drugs would be required to be effective—more than are necessary to prevent rejection of a transplanted human organ. As these large doses would also suppress the body's immune response to invading bacteria and viruses, the patient would be at an increased risk of infection and other drug-related complications.

Although there are few experimental data on which to base a conclusion, chronic rejection like that occurring after allografting is known to occur after transplantation between closely related species. Since there is a much greater discrepancy between the donor and recipient tissue types than between two humans, we would anticipate that chronic rejection would develop earlier and progress more aggressively in an animal organ than in a human organ. The experimental data we have to date suggest that this is indeed the case.

Transplantation between distantly related animals

The first barrier: hyperacute rejection

When a widely disparate animal species (for example, the pig) is used as the donor of an organ to a primate, an even more rapid destruction of the transplanted organ occurs. Pioneering work in the 1960s and 1970s by several groups, particularly by University of Minnesota surgeons John Najarian (Figure 5.1) and Robert Perper, demonstrated that this hyperacute rejection is caused by the presence of antibodies *already circulating* in large numbers in the recipient's blood (Figure 5.2). Humans, apes, and baboons all have antibodies directed against pig tissues, and these can also destroy organs from other species, such as the sheep and cow. Humans (and other primates) are therefore naturally sensitized against the pig.

These antibodies do not come from consuming pork; they are found even in people who have never eaten pork in their lives. The reason for these antibodies is that the pig has an antigen, or sugar molecule, on the internal lining of its blood vessels that is identical to those found on the surface of certain bacteria, viruses, and parasites. Although we have no antibodies against this particular sugar when we are born, our gut becomes colonized by a large number of microorganisms as soon as we start to eat and drink.

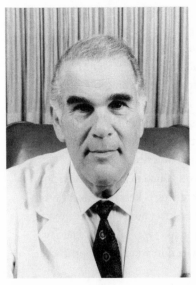

figure 5.1. *University of Minnesota transplant surgeon John Najarian, who, with Robert Perper, determined that the hyperacute rejection of a widely disparate xenografted organ was initiated by an antibody-mediated attack. (Courtesy of John Najarian, M.D.)*

figure 5.2. *Hyperacute rejection of a pig organ transplanted in a patient frequently occurs within minutes. It ensues after antibodies bind to the linear sugar chains lining pig blood vessels. This antibody-antigen interaction activates complement, which destroys the pig tissues.*

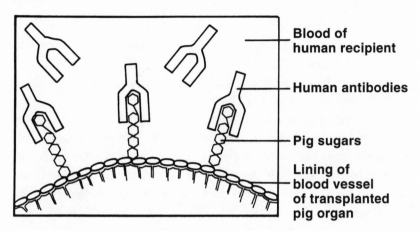

Blood of human recipient

Human antibodies

Pig sugars

Lining of blood vessel of transplanted pig organ

To protect ourselves against infection, we develop antibodies against certain of these organisms. In cases where these sugar molecules happen, by chance, to be common to both the microorganisms and to the pig, the resulting antibodies will not only destroy these bacteria but will destroy pig organs and tissues as well. This unfortunate coincidence means that, from a very early age, we are naturally primed to destroy pig tissues if and when they are transplanted into our body. (Fortunately, the antibodies have no effect if pork is digested in the bowel and its constituent parts absorbed through the gut wall.)

After transplantation of a pig organ into a human or nonhuman primate, these antibodies, which are circulating in the blood at all times, immediately bind to the antigens on the surface of the pig blood vessels (Figure 5.2). This antibody-antigen binding triggers a complex cascade of proteins known as the complement cascade, which is what causes the destruction of the pig organ. It is a dramatic and rapid sequence of events—the efficient defense mechanism meant to knock out microscopic invaders that would make us ill instead destroys the transplanted organ within minutes.

The nature of anti-pig antibodies. Although medical scientists have known since the 1960s that humans and other primates have antibodies against pig tissues, it wasn't until the 1990s that we identified the exact target of these antibodies, namely, a certain sugar molecule. This discovery was made by a collaborating team of scientists and surgeons from Oklahoma City, Oklahoma (of which one of us was a member), and from Edmonton, Alberta, and was reported at the First International Congress on Xenotransplantation held in Minneapolis in 1991.

The manner in which the target sugar was identified was relatively simple. Because antibodies are found in plasma (blood from which the red and white blood cells and other cellular elements have been removed), human plasma containing the anti-pig antibodies was perfused through the blood vessels of several kidneys and hearts that had been removed from pigs. The antibodies in the plasma attached themselves to the unknown sugars on the lining of the pig blood vessels. The remainder of the plasma passed freely through the organ and was discarded. The anti-pig antibodies that had stuck to the pig blood vessel walls were then released (eluted) by flushing the pig organ with a chemical that breaks the bond between the antibody and the sugar antigen. The eluted antibodies were collected and tested in the laboratory against a large panel of known sugars. The sugar was identified as a form of galactose (often abbreviated to Gal), which is not very different in structure from glucose, a type of sugar that is important to the body as a source of energy. Although there are many different forms of galactose, the anti-pig antibodies were found to be very specific, binding only to a galactose sugar in which the two terminal molecules are joined at a very specific site, designated as an α-1–3 linkage. Remarkably, a different form of galactose with a very small change in the structure of the sugar is not a target for the anti-pig antibodies.

The discovery that it is antibodies directed specifically against Gal sugar antigens that initiate hyperacute rejection—made by a small group of investigators including Croatian medical scientist Eugen Koren, of the Oklahoma Medical Research Foundation, who carried out the isolation of the anti-pig antibodies, and Canadian biochemist Heather Good, who tested the antibodies against the panel of sugars—has proved to be an important one. It has enabled us to develop methods of removing these anti-Gal antibodies from the potential human recipient and also of exploring the possibility of genetically engineering a pig that no longer expresses the troublesome Gal sugar on its blood vessels. Although these therapeutic efforts are discussed in later chapters, suffice it to say at this stage that we believe that if we can prevent the binding of the anti-pig antibody to the Gal sugar, then the complement cascade will not be set in motion and the pig organ will not be destroyed. Hyperacute rejection will be stopped in its tracks.

Hoping to avoid the need for genetic engineering, the Oklahoma City group, in collaboration with Parisian immunogeneticist Rafael Oriol, searched for a potential donor animal that does not express the Gal sugar on its blood vessels. But Gal is present on the lining of the blood vessels of all non-primate mammals, including all of those that might be suitable as organ donors for humans, such as the cow, sheep, and goat. The only Gal-negative species appear to be birds, reptiles, and the capybara, which is the world's largest rodent. This is certainly not a promising group of potential organ donors, although two young surgeons who spent time working with one of us in Oklahoma, Shigeki Taniguchi and Yong Ye, investigated the potential of the ostrich heart. Unfortunately, they found that not only did it not beat well when its nerve supply was divided, but there were other sugars on its blood vessels against which humans also appear to have antibodies.

Uri Galili, biological detective.   Those interested in evolution will be intrigued to learn that it is only humans, great apes, and Old World monkeys that have antibodies directed against the Gal sugar (Figure 5.3). New World monkeys and all lower nonprimate mammals, including Australasian marsupials, actually make the sugar and express it on their tissues. They therefore do not make the antibodies, since only in autoimmune disease states do animals make antibodies directed against their own tissues. From extensive biological detective work by Israeli scientist Uri Galili, now based in the United States, and others, we know that even humans and the higher non-human primates have the gene that encodes the enzyme that makes the Gal sugar, but in us, unlike in the pig, the gene is now nonfunctional.

Uri Galili, who was the first to describe the existence of anti-Gal antibodies in humans, has hypothesized that this evolutionary change could have been in response to an unknown lethal microorganism that expressed the Gal sugar. Perhaps only those primates with naturally low (or even no) levels of Gal survived, since they were able to make anti-Gal antibodies to destroy the invading bacteria or viruses. Those primates that could not manufacture anti-Gal antibodies died from the infection. (The infection presumably did not affect pigs and other lower mammals, as they retained Gal production and did not need to produce anti-Gal antibodies.) Of course, the exact biological events that occurred are unknown, but, as New World monkeys still express the Gal sugar, whatever happened must have occurred after the separation of Old World monkeys from New World monkeys, which has been estimated to have taken place between 30 million and 40 million years ago (Figure 5.3).

This significant difference between Old and New World monkeys was used to demonstrate the unique importance of the presence of the Gal epitope (the specific molecular feature that elicits the antibody response) in the

figure 5.3. *Evolutionary time scale of mammals during the past 125 million years. All mammals originally synthesized the Gal sugar, which was made by the enzyme α-1, 3-galactosyltransferase (GT). Evidence suggests that approximately 10 million to 25 million years ago the Old World higher primates were afflicted by a lethal infection caused by a microorganism that also expressed the Gal sugar. Only those primates that could produce anti-Gal antibodies survived. This necessitated suppression of the synthesis of the Gal sugar by mutation of the gene for the enzyme GT. (Modified from U. Galili,* Science and Medicine, *5, 28–37, 1998.)*

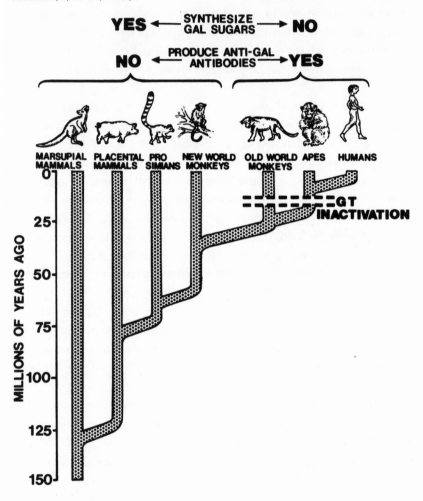

donor organ. Monkeys, whether from the Old or New World, are genetically extremely close. (A glance at Table 10.2 will confirm their close evolutionary relationship.) One would anticipate that organ transplants between them would be rejected by a mechanism not dissimilar to that which occurs with chimpanzee-to-human transplants; certainly, hyperacute rejection would not be anticipated. But, as demonstrated by immunologist Jeff Platt's group at Duke University in North Carolina, New World monkey hearts transplanted into Old World baboons are indeed rejected hyperacutely. The presence of Gal molecules on the New World monkey organ and anti-Gal antibodies in the baboon overrides all of the similarities between the two species.

We are steadily gaining more and more information on the nature of the hyperacute rejection that occurs when a pig organ is transplanted into a human or baboon. The major destructive effect is by the complement cascade proteins (the proteins are often called *complement* for short, and we speak of "activating complement"), but there are other mechanisms that are also involved. The cells that line the pig blood vessels are probably activated by the anti-Gal antibodies, and this brings about significant changes in the cells. One important change is that these cells lose their ability to prevent blood clots from forming on their surface. This increased tendency for clot formation is probably a major contributing factor to the blockage that occurs in the small blood vessels of the transplanted pig organ.

Of one thing we are certain: none of the immunosuppressive drugs currently available to us, even when combined with one another in large doses, is at all successful in preventing hyperacute rejection. They have no effect on the activity of antibodies or complement. We therefore have to come up with completely new forms of therapy and new approaches if we are to overcome hyperacute rejection. Our attempts to do so are discussed in subsequent chapters.

The remaining barriers: peeling the onion

What happens if hyperacute rejection can be prevented? Although this question has been on the minds of transplant scientists for many years, we were unable to get past this barrier until recently. Scientists have now been able to prevent hyperacute rejection by various methods, most notably by the use of techniques that significantly reduce antibody levels, or by using agents that deplete the body's supply of complement or prevent complement activation. Biotechnology companies have also been able to genetically engineer pigs that are resistant to human complement. In these various ways, we have begun to gain information on what happens when hyperacute rejection is overcome.

Unfortunately, evidence is accumulating that indicates that when one immune barrier has been overcome, there is another waiting. Indeed, unraveling the mysteries of the human body's response to a transplanted pig organ has been likened to peeling an onion. As soon as one layer has been peeled off, another is revealed. This analogy of the onion can be carried further in that, after the painstaking work to peel off one layer, the realization that there are perhaps several layers remaining is frequently accompanied by tears. (However, as Tom Starzl has written, "Only those who have known complete despair can understand the full meaning of jubilation.")

When hyperacute rejection is prevented, rejection still takes place within a few days, in a form not dissimilar to that which occurs when transplants are performed between closely related animal species. This is almost certainly related to the increased production of anti-pig antibodies, but is probably not caused by complement. Other mechanisms are involved that are still not fully understood. Certain white blood cells, such as NK cells and macrophages, are attracted to the pig organ, possibly by the presence of the antibodies that have become bound to the cell surface antigens, and help in the destruction of the organ.

If this form of rejection can in turn be prevented or overcome, then we are likely to see cellular rejection similar to that which occurs after human organ transplants. As yet, however, we have very little information on this because few therapeutic approaches have been able to protect pig organs from the recipient's anti-pig antibodies for a sufficient length of time. In the meantime, we can guess that because the tissue type of the pig is so different from that of the human, the cellular rejection of pig organs may well prove to be aggressive and severe.

We remain unsure as to which pharmacologic agents, if any, will be most efficient in preventing the cellular rejection of a pig organ. A combination of agents will almost certainly be essential, and we may even have to await development of new types of drugs that are not yet currently available. Some scientists involved in this aspect of xenotransplantation research believe that the cellular response to a pig organ may be so severe that none of our drugs, even in combination, will be sufficiently powerful to prevent it unless given in prohibitively large doses that result in major problems. If true, this would be ultimately frustrating, since many of us currently believe that if we can successfully overcome the initial antibody-mediated problems of xenografting, the most important hurdle will be behind us.

To date, no transplanted pig organ has survived long enough in a monkey, baboon, or human to determine whether chronic rejection will develop. It is almost inconceivable, however, that chronic rejection—like that seen in long-surviving human transplanted organs—will not occur. Indeed, it is more likely that chronic rejection will develop earlier in a xenograft than in an allograft, reflecting the greater disparity between the human and pig. If, despite successfully overcoming antibody-mediated and cellular rejection, organ failure occurs from chronic rejection within a few months, xenotransplantation might not be a viable clinical option until ways are also developed to overcome this problem. However, if chronic rejection develops over years, rather than months, then retransplantation is always an option available to us. The great advantage of using the pig is that there will never be a shortage of suitable donor organs.

The immunological barriers to xenotransplantation are considerable. In the next few chapters we shall explore how ingenious scientists and surgeons are attempting to overcome them.

chapter 6

A Spoonful of Sugar

Preventing rejection

The Scientist as Guinea Pig ○ ○ ○

The incomparable ingenuity of the human race is exemplified in the variety of methods currently being tested in laboratories around the world in attempts to overcome the violent destruction that occurs immediately after transplantation of an animal organ. Many of these efforts are innovative, but perhaps no researcher has been as courageous in testing his theories as Venezuelan medical scientist Egidio Romano. Romano's initial interest was in antibodies that destroy human red blood cells rather than transplanted animal organs, but his work had implications for xenotransplantation.

We can chemically synthesize sugars that mimic the sugars present on human red blood cells. Romano and his colleagues believed that if such sugars were injected into a patient, they would be bound by antibodies directed against that sugar. The antibodies would therefore be "immobilized" and could no longer attack the patient's own red blood cells. To test this theory, he and his colleagues initially injected the hitherto untested synthetic sugars into their own veins to check on their safety and toxicity. Fortunately, they all survived this experience.

But we get ahead of ourselves; Romano's story comes a little later in this chapter. In this and the following two chapters we shall discuss the special problems relating to the use of the pig as a donor, and review some of the exciting efforts being made to overcome the rapid rejection of transplanted pig organs.

The Challenge Facing Us o o o

We have to develop treatments designed to overcome or prevent the various types of rejection—antibody-mediated, cellular, and chronic—that can potentially occur when a pig organ is transplanted into a human recipient. The well-respected Stanford transplant immunologist Randall Morris is a popular lecturer, partly because of the humor he injects into his scientific presentations. He has a slide that he projects that states: "There are three golden rules for achieving successful transplantation." As his audience waits expectantly, he rapidly follows with another slide: "Unfortunately, we don't know any of them." The same could be said for xenotransplantation. However, although we may not have any golden rules, we are rapidly learning how we can achieve survival of animal organ grafts in humans.

Most research attention to date has been directed toward overcoming hyperacute rejection, as this is the first major obstacle to successful xenotransplantation. If we cannot get over this hurdle, we will never face the subsequent hurdles.

Overcoming the First Barrier: Preventing Hyperacute Rejection o o o

Two quite different approaches can be taken, and it is possible that these two approaches may need to be combined if we are to be successful. Therapy can be aimed at either the potential recipient or the potential donor. Therapies aimed at the recipient entail methods of depleting the recipient of anti-pig antibodies, of inhibiting the antibody from binding to the pig antigens, of depleting the recipient of stores of complement, or of inhibiting the function of complement.

Therapies aimed at the donor require the genetic engineering of a pig that either does not express the usual Gal sugar on its blood vessels (and thus has no target for the anti-pig antibodies) or expresses molecules that inhibit the complement attack of the human host.

We shall here consider only therapies aimed at modifying the immune response of the human recipient. Approaches to modifying the donor pig by genetic engineering techniques will be reviewed in the next chapter.

Depletion or inhibition of anti-pig antibodies

For many years we have known from experimental studies that if the potential human (or nonhuman primate) recipient's blood is perfused through an isolated pig organ, then the recipient's anti-pig antibodies bind to the sugar antigens lining the blood vessels of the pig organ. If this perfusion continues for an hour or two (often requiring two or more sequential pig organs if the first is rapidly rejected) then the anti-pig antibodies are totally depleted from the potential recipient. If another pig organ is then immediately transplanted into the recipient, it survives much longer than if transplanted into a recipient in which antibody has not been depleted.

In experiments performed by our research group when we were based in Cape Town several years ago, the blood of a recipient baboon was perfused through a pair of pig kidneys for a couple of hours. This was immediately followed by transplantation of the heart from the same pig into the baboon. The heart survived for five days, even though no immunosuppressive drug therapy was given. This was in contrast to the usual survival of a pig heart in a baboon of a few minutes to two or three hours at most.

The depletion of anti-pig antibodies has also been confirmed in three human volunteers in Britain and Sweden, all patients on renal dialysis who agreed to have their blood perfused through pig kidneys. Hyperacute rejection can therefore be prevented by this relatively simple method, but unfortunately the effect is only temporary, with anti-pig antibodies returning within a few days.

Refining the technique: plasma exchange

There are numerous ways of refining this rather crude, though effective, technique of depletion of anti-pig antibodies. One such refinement is plasma exchange. As the blood is withdrawn from the body of the recipient, it is passed through a device that separates the cellular constituents of the blood from the remaining plasma. As humans can manufacture antibodies against every conceivable antigen (that is, against almost anything foreign which enters the body), the plasma contains large numbers of different antibodies, not only anti-pig antibodies. Instead of being returned to the body, this separated plasma can be discarded and replaced by another suitable fluid, such as a salt solution (saline) or protein solution (albumin). If saline or albumin (instead of the plasma) is returned to the body together with the cellular components, then the blood is temporarily depleted of *all* antibodies.

If the above procedure is combined with the administration of immunosuppressive drugs, the production of new anti-pig antibodies (as well as all other antibodies) is partially suppressed. Similarly, there is some evidence that, if the recipient's spleen is removed—the spleen being a major store of the B cells that produce antibodies—antibody rebound can also be reduced. But if plasma exchange is not continued on a regular and frequent basis, antibodies of all sorts slowly but steadily return; this is because no combination of immunosuppressive drugs is successful in suppressing B cell activity completely.

Plasma exchange is used successfully in this way in the treatment of certain diseases, where the aim is to remove antibodies from the blood. However, because it depletes the body of all antibodies even though removal of only one may be required, the patient no longer has antibodies that protect against infecting organisms. Although these antibodies are manufactured anew within a few days of cessation of plasma exchange therapy, the patient is clearly at increased risk for infection during the period that the antibodies are depleted.

Being more specific: depleting anti-Gal antibodies

Since the nature of the pig antigens against which human anti-pig antibodies are directed was identified as being the Gal sugar, we have been able to refine this form of depletion therapy. Following the separation of cells from plasma, we can now remove only the anti-Gal antibodies from the plasma, returning all other antibodies to the patient. To achieve this, the plasma is circulated through a container filled with the specific synthetic Gal sugar. The anti-pig antibodies bind to the sugar, and the plasma steadily becomes depleted of these antibodies alone, leaving all beneficial antibodies to be returned to the patient. Pig hearts in baboon recipients depleted of anti-Gal antibodies in this way survive for several days.

Although these techniques can now routinely prevent hyperacute rejection—a significant step in the right direction—we have been unable to completely prevent the slow production of antibodies by the B cells. When the antibody level rises high enough, usually within days, rejection of the transplanted organ occurs. There is some hope, however, that if the anti-pig antibodies can be depleted for a sufficient period of time—possibly two to three weeks—there is a chance that when they do return, they will not bring about rejection. The recipient would then be said to have "accommodated" to the presence of the organ.

Although accommodation has been well-documented in several rodent organ transplantation models, it remains a poorly understood process. Harvard immunologist Fritz Bach and his group have provided data that suggest that changes occur in gene expression in the cells of the donor organ and that these protect them from destruction.

"Accommodating" the transplanted organ: lessons from blood group incompatibilities

What is the evidence that accommodation may take place and allow the long-term functioning of a pig organ in a human? What evidence there is comes mainly from experience with the transplantation of a human organ from a patient of one blood type into a patient of another (incompatible) blood type.

There are four blood groups: A, B, AB, and O (Table 6.1). To say that someone has type A blood means that on the surface of that person's red blood cells, *but also on the lining of all of the blood vessels throughout the person's body,* there is a sugar with a structure designated as A. People who lack the A sugar on their red blood cells and blood vessels (that is, individuals of blood types O or B) develop antibodies against the A sugar (anti-A antibodies). If an organ is taken from an individual of blood type A and transplanted into another individual who is not of blood group A or AB, then that organ has a high chance of being rejected hyperacutely because of the presence of the anti-A antibodies in the recipient. An organ from a blood group B donor would likely be rejected if transplanted into a recipient of blood type A or O, as humans of these groups make anti-B antibodies.

With very rare exceptions, none of us, no matter what our blood type, has antibodies against O sugars. Therefore, blood or an organ can be donated by a blood type O individual to any recipient, irrespective of the recipient's blood type. Conversely, individuals of blood group AB, who express both A and B sugars on their red blood cells and blood vessels, develop neither anti-A nor anti-B antibodies and are therefore universal recipients, that is, they can accept a blood transfusion or an organ transplant from any donor, irrespective of the donor's blood type.

The hyperacute rejection that occurs when an organ is transplanted across this ABO barrier is almost identical to the reaction that occurs when a pig organ is transplanted into a human. The initiating factor is the presence

table 6.1

Relationship of Blood Group Antigens and Antibodies in Humans

Antibodies[a]	Antigens[b]			
	O	A	B	AB
Anti-A	+	−	+	−
Anti-B	+	+	−	−

For example, a subject who expresses either the O or B antigen will develop antibodies against the A antigen.

[a] Antibodies are present in human plasma.
[b] Antigens are present on the red blood cells and on the lining of blood vessels throughout the body.

of antibodies in the recipient (in this case anti-A or anti-B rather than anti-Gal) that bind to the equivalent sugars on the surface of the donor organ, leading to activation of complement and the rapid destruction of the transplanted organ.

In humans, a transplanted ABO-incompatible organ has an approximately 60% chance of undergoing hyperacute rejection. Why the remaining 40% of recipients do not reject an incompatible ABO organ remains unknown. If we could determine the exact reason for this phenomenon, then we might be in a position to modify the immune response of all recipients to ensure that an ABO-incompatible organ is always accepted. Knowledge of how we could do this might also give us a clue as to how we could overcome rejection of pig organs by humans.

The pioneering work of Guy Alexandre

In the 1970s and 1980s, a surgical team in Brussels headed by Belgian surgeon Guy Alexandre was carrying out kidney transplants from living donors who were close relatives of the patient. Because of the close genetic relationship, there was usually a good HLA (white blood cell) tissue match between the potential recipient and the potential donor. Such closely matched organ transplants generally function extremely well for many years. However, in some of these cases, although there was a good tissue match, there was a mismatch (or incompatibility) of ABO blood type.

Guy Alexandre and his colleagues decided to perform plasma exchange on the potential recipients. They removed the plasma (containing, for example, the anti-A antibodies) and replaced it with saline or another innocuous solution that did not contain any antibodies. Alexandre coupled this with removing the spleen from the potential recipient and administering immunosuppressive drugs. When the antibody level was zero or close to zero, he transplanted the ABO-incompatible donor kidney into the recipient.

In the great majority of cases, even when the antibody returned, the organ was not rejected. Some of these organs have now been functioning in healthy recipients for over 10 years. In other words, accommodation has taken place. We now have a healthy patient who has a well-functioning transplanted kidney that expresses a sugar against which that same patient has specific antibodies. These antibodies should theoretically rapidly destroy the organ, and yet rejection has not taken place. The explanation for this phenomenon remains uncertain.

Will accommodation take place after pig organ transplantation?

The similarity between transplantation of a human organ into an ABO-incompatible patient and placement of a pig organ into a human recipient is obvious and leads us to be optimistic that accommodation of a pig organ may also occur under the right conditions. But we do not yet know this for certain. Although there are now reports of survival of pig hearts and kidneys in monkeys or baboons for periods over two months, there has been no definite evidence that accommodation has occurred.

There are, however, several significant differences between ABO-incompatible human-to-human allografting and pig-to-human xenotransplantation. First, humans have a much greater quantity of antibodies directed against the Gal sugar than they do against A or B sugars. This may be very important. Second, in the ABO-incompatible situation, the complement that causes destruction of the organ graft in the unmodified recipient is from the same species as the donor. We know that a human organ has a large degree of protection against human complement, provided by complement-regulatory proteins on the lining of the blood vessels of the organs. As hyperacute rejection of a transplanted human organ can occur under certain conditions, the protection provided by these complement-regulatory proteins is clearly not always effective, but it does work under most circumstances. Pig organs, on the other hand, express pig complement-regulatory proteins, which similarly prevent damage by pig complement. However, those proteins give pig organs little protection against *human* complement.

Because of these and other differences, accommodation may be difficult, or even impossible, to achieve in pig-to-human transplants. If so, we will have to find some method of maintaining the recipient's anti-pig antibodies at extremely low or nonexistent levels in the long term—maybe forever. Although this will be exceedingly difficult, it may not be impossible.

Egidio Romano's new concept: antibody inhibition by injected sugars

A second approach to protecting the transplanted organ from the antibody response of the potential recipient has also evolved from work in studying ABO incompatibility. In 1987, Egidio Romano put forward the concept that, rather than remove the antibodies, they could equally well be inhibited or neutralized by infusing the relevant synthetic sugar into the blood (Figure 6.1). His concept was that, for example, anti-A antibodies would bind to the infused synthetic A sugar and would therefore no longer be free to attack a subsequently transplanted A-type organ.

His initial interest in this topic was not in relation to organ transplantation but to the treatment of newborn babies with a condition known as

figure 6.1. *The infusion into the patient's blood of synthetic linear Gal sugars that mimic those on the pig organs leads to binding of the synthetic sugars by the patient's anti-pig antibodies, which are then immobilized and inhibited from binding to the Gal sugars lining the blood vessels of a subsequently transplanted pig organ. (Compare with figure 5.2, p. 63.) As a result, complement is not activated.*

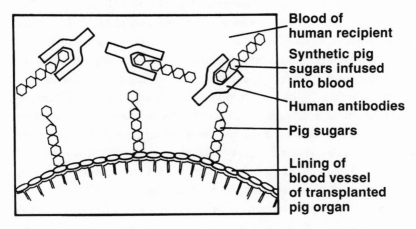

Blood of
human recipient

Synthetic pig
sugars infused
into blood

Human antibodies

Pig sugars

Lining of
blood vessel
of transplanted
pig organ

ABO hemolytic disease of the newborn. In severe cases, this condition, caused by the presence of maternal antibodies against the fetus's red blood cells, can result in brain damage or even death.

As a preliminary step, Romano injected the A and B synthetic sugars into himself and other members of his research team to ensure that there were no toxic effects that might harm the babies. He then went on to treat a number of newborn babies suffering from this condition. He was able to demonstrate that the injury to the babies' red blood cells caused by the antibodies could be prevented or significantly reduced. With no or little destruction of their red blood cells, the babies survived unharmed. This is typical of some of the ingenious, yet unheralded, investigations being carried out by dedicated scientists in countries not generally associated with medical or scientific research.

Following this important study, in which Romano proved the concept that sugars injected intravenously could inhibit or neutralize anti-sugar antibodies, our group in Oklahoma collaborated with him and others to see whether the infusion of the respective sugars (AB or Gal) would prevent the hyperacute rejection of ABO-incompatible allografts or pig xenografts in baboons. The infusion of the sugar into the baboon's blood successfully prevented hyperacute rejection of ABO-incompatible baboon organs, but was less successful at protecting transplanted pig organs.

Therapy at $1 million a day

The synthesis of these sugars, whether they are human A or B sugars or pig Gal sugars, has until recently been an expensive and time-consuming procedure. The A and B sugars used in our own studies were produced by a small Canadian biotechnology company, Chembiomed Ltd., and were commercially available to blood transfusion laboratories to be used for blood typing purposes. They were sold at a cost of U.S. $90 per milligram of sugar. In our own experience, in order to fully neutralize a baboon's anti-A or anti-B antibody, we needed to infuse approximately 500 mg of sugar each hour— in other words, if we had had to purchase it commercially, approximately $45,000 worth of sugar each hour! Several of the baboons received a continuous infusion of sugar for up to two weeks—using almost $1 million worth of sugar each day! (The reader may consider it not totally incoincidental to learn that Chembiomed subsequently went out of business when the provincial government discontinued its financial support.)

Today, however, with improvements in technology in both the synthetic and the newer enzymatic techniques, production is becoming much less expensive. One of the leaders in this field in the United States is a Philadelphia biotechology company, Neose, Inc., one of whose senior staff estimates that if intravenous infusion therapy could be shown to be successful for xeno-transplantation and began to be used on a large scale, such sugars might eventually be able to be produced for perhaps as little as a few cents per milligram, which would make such therapy a much more realistic therapeutic approach.

The difference in the amount of Gal sugar required for intravenous infusion when compared with that required for the circulation of plasma through a Gal-filled cartridge (as described earlier) is illustrated by the fact that only 25 mg is required to fill a container (which is reusable), whereas almost 500 times this amount (12 g) is required for each 24 hours of infusion in a 15-kg (33-lb) baboon, and several days' continuous infusion is necessary. Larger amounts would, of course, be necessary for a human weighing four or five times as much.

Research using baboons

We have alluded to the important information obtained by carrying out auxiliary heart transplantation in a baboon. It is unfortunate that any animals have to be used in medical research, especially baboons, but the fact that it is only humans and nonhuman primates that have anti-Gal antibodies virtually necessitates research into xenotransplantation being performed in baboons rather than in lower species. Similarly, it is only humans and nonhuman primates who have equivalent anti-ABO antibodies. To those who would like to see animal experimentation kept to an absolute minimum, which in our experience is the wish of the majority of those involved in medical research, it should be emphasized that transplantation of a pig heart as an auxiliary pump is a relatively minor operation for the recipient baboon. If the auxiliary heart is rejected, which usually occurs without any ill effects to the baboon, it is removed (again under anesthesia). The baboon can then be returned to the baboon colony to continue life as normal (or as normal as is possible in captivity). Undoubtedly the baboon experiences some discomfort. As with many other aspects of life, however, the experimenter—indeed, society in general—is faced with weighing the relative harm to one party (on this occasion, the baboon) against the potential benefits to another party (the human race).

A taste of its own medicine: manufacturing antibodies against antibodies

The concept of inhibiting anti-pig antibodies by introducing intravenous synthetic sugars that "compete" for antibody with the sugars on the surface of the transplanted organ can be utilized in another way. Antibodies are protein structures manufactured in the body, and it is possible to make antibodies against antibodies. This can be done by injecting human (or baboon) anti-pig antibodies into a mouse. The mouse recognizes the protein antibodies as being foreign, and manufactures antibodies against them. Such antibodies directed against other antibodies are called anti-idiotypic antibodies, or AIAs. Using various techniques, these AIAs can be produced in large amounts, sufficient to inject back into a human (or baboon). After intravenous injection, the AIA binds to the anti-pig antibody, which is thus inhibited or neutralized in just the same way as when it binds to an infused synthetic Gal sugar. The strength of binding between an antibody and an AIA is generally stronger than between an antibody and a sugar, and such AIAs may therefore protect a transplanted pig organ more efficiently than will a soluble sugar. The first such AIAs produced against human anti-pig antibodies were made in mice by Eugen Koren and his colleagues in Oklahoma City. Largely through the work of a young South African scientist named Francisca Neethling, they were demonstrated to greatly reduce the antibody-mediated destruction of pig cells by baboon anti-pig antibodies. Work is continuing in this field.

Depletion or inhibition of complement

Although it is the antibody that initiates the process that destroys the transplanted pig organ in hyperacute rejection, it is complement—a complex sequence of proteins in the blood—that actually carries out the destruction. Several groups have concentrated their attention not on the antibody-antigen part of the process but on depleting the amount of complement in the recipient or inhibiting its activity.

The venom of the cobra

One agent that causes complement depletion is a toxin found in the venom of cobra snakes. When purified as cobra venom factor (CVF) and injected intravenously or intramuscularly into a human or nonhuman primate, the toxin causes rapid consumption—and therefore depletion—of the existing complement in the blood. (As might be expected of a snake venom, CVF can be fatal if given in excess. However, purification reduces the toxic effects and makes it safe to use in the prescribed dose.) After its administration, it takes several days for the complement level to return to normal. As early as the 1960s, several groups documented that, if a pig organ is transplanted during a period of complement depletion, then organ survival is prolonged until the complement returns to a sufficient level to once again be destructive. If repeated injections of CVF are administered over the course of a number of days, then complement depletion is maintained and graft survival is prolonged further, particularly if combined with immunosuppressive drug therapy.

In our own laboratory in Oklahoma City, Takaaki Kobayashi, a young surgeon from Nagoya in Japan, extended pig heart survival in a baboon for up to 25 days in one experiment. At that time, it was the longest survival of a pig organ ever achieved in a primate. However, when we looked at tissue samples taken from the pig heart during that period, we found that as early as the first week after the transplant, microscopic changes were taking place that were suggestive of antibody-mediated rejection. The presence of anti-pig antibody (which was not affected by the CVF) appeared to be causing slow rejection in the absence of complement, even though hyperacute rejection had been prevented. We concluded, therefore, that depletion or inhibition of complement alone might not be sufficient to totally prevent rejection. Work from other centers has also indicated that it is likely to prove essential to deplete or inhibit anti-pig antibody as well as complement. Nevertheless, CVF is proving a valuable adjunct in several experimental models of xenotransplantation.

Soluble complement receptor 1

Several other approaches are being investigated to deplete or inhibit complement. Complement attaches to receptors on the transplanted pig organ cells, one of which is known as complement receptor 1. These receptors can be produced in a soluble form that has been named soluble complement receptor 1 (sCR1). When sCR1 is injected into the blood, the complement binds to it and is therefore prevented from binding to the complement receptors on a transplanted organ. (One can see similarity between this therapeutic approach and that devised by Egidio Romano, in which the Gal sugar was injected into the blood to inhibit anti-pig antibody.) Therapy with sCR1 in xenotransplantation has been investigated at several centers, in particular by a group at the Johns Hopkins University Hospital in Baltimore, headed by pathologist Fred Sanfilippo. When administered to a monkey, together with high doses of immunosuppressive therapy, sCR1 has extended pig heart transplant survival to over 40 days.

There are other drugs that also inhibit complement activity by various mechanisms, but to date these have not proved as effective as CVF or sCR1.

Overcoming the Second Barrier:
Preventing Delayed Antibody-Mediated Rejection o o o

Though we can avoid hyperacute rejection through a number of therapeutic strategies, a form of antibody-mediated rejection eventually develops, suggesting that the presence of anti-pig antibody alone (without complement, which we can deplete or inhibit for weeks at a time) may be sufficient to lead to this event. Other factors may also play roles, though they are too complex and numerous to discuss here. Research into these factors is underway at several centers, particularly by immunologists Fritz Bach, at the Beth Israel-Deaconess Medical Center in Boston, and Jeff Platt, formerly at Duke University and now at the Mayo Clinic in Minnesota. Current evidence suggests that because anti-pig antibody may play a major role, it is essential to work on minimizing the effect of that antibody, at least during the early days after a pig organ is transplanted.

Given the current difficulties that face us in trying to overcome this delayed response, it seems almost certain that a combination of therapies will be required. One small but welcome sign is that this delayed rejection has been suppressed, at least temporarily, in experiments in which very high doses of immunosuppressive drugs were administered to recipient monkeys. Although such high drug doses were poorly tolerated by the monkeys, and would be unlikely to be tolerated by human recipients, the study did illustrate that, even in the presence of anti-pig antibody, rejection could be suppressed for a period of time. (As the great 18th-century French physician Alexis Littre said, "It is often sufficient to know, in the large, that a thing may be possible.") These studies, carried out in Cambridge, in the United Kingdom, suggest that if the right immunosuppressive drug combination can be identified and anti-pig antibodies are maintained at low levels, perhaps this delayed form of antibody-mediated rejection can be prevented completely.

Overcoming the Third Barrier:
Preventing Acute Cellular Rejection ○ ○ ○

If the problems caused by antibody and complement can be successfully overcome, it seems inevitable that a third phase of rejection, acute cellular rejection, will attack the transplanted pig organ. Physicians involved in the care of transplant patients are very familiar with acute cellular rejection, as it affects most human organs transplanted into patients today. It tends to occur relatively quickly after the transplant, most commonly within the first three months, but if successfully treated, as it usually can be, it becomes less of a problem with the passage of time. Indeed, it is relatively rare after the first post-transplant year. The recipient's body slowly acclimates to the new organ and becomes more tolerant of its presence. In a sense, the early immune response burns itself out and the body accepts the newcomer with less hostility than at first. Nevertheless, if the amount of immunosuppressive therapy that the patient is receiving is reduced too much, an acute cellular rejection episode can occur in most patients even many years after the transplant operation.

Just how severe cellular rejection of a pig organ will be remains uncertain; we have rarely successfully overcome the earlier antibody-mediated rejection to allow a pig organ to survive long enough to be subjected to the body's cellular attack. We therefore have to rely on information gleaned from less reliable sources, such as laboratory work with pig cells and data from experiments in rodents. In mice, for example, it has been possible to concoct experiments where this form of rejection can be studied.

In the early days of exploration into xenotransplantation, researchers hoped that the cellular response to organs from a very different species, such as the pig, would be weak—certainly weaker than to an allograft. This opinion was based on experiments that suggested that the cells involved in the human immune attack, largely the T lymphocytes, would either not recognize cells from a species that was so distant from the human or would be unable to mount a good response, again because of the differences between the two species. However, this original optimism would seem to be misplaced. With the increasing amounts of data becoming available from laboratories around the world, it now looks as if cellular rejection of a pig organ may be at least as strong as that of a human organ. In the Cambridge pig-to-monkey experiments referred to above, however, intensive immunosuppressive therapy administered in an attempt to prevent antibody-mediated rejection, although not fully successful in this respect, does appear to have prevented acute cellular rejection. This observation is a cause for cautious optimism.

Anti-rejection drugs

In cellular rejection, the T cells of the host actually invade the transplanted organ and take steps to destroy it. This attack can be prevented or reversed by drugs that either kill the T cells or at least block the production of the chemicals they produce, such as cytokines, which can injure the transplanted organ. Until fairly recently, there were relatively few drugs available to us, but during the past five years or so two more potent ones have come on to the market after long periods of research.

The original drug commonly used after organ transplantation, introduced largely by British transplant surgeon Sir Roy Calne in the early 1960s, is still being used on a daily basis. However, this drug, known as azathioprine, is steadily being replaced by newer, more potent agents. Azathioprine is one of a family of cytotoxic drugs, several of which are used in the treatment of cancer, that kill cells while they are dividing to form new cells. What both cancer cells and the T cells involved in rejection have in common is that they are both dividing rapidly, one to increase the size of the tumor and the other to develop an army to reject the foreign organ. Azathioprine therefore kills the T lymphocytes rather than all of the other cells in the body, though there is a danger it will do just that if given in too high a dosage. Generally, however, it is an easy and relatively safe drug to use (Table 6.2).

For many years the only support azathioprine received was from the corticosteroid drugs, which are used in the treatment of many disorders, including arthritis and asthma. Steroids have numerous effects on the immune system, some of which are still poorly understood, but the bottom line as far as organ transplantation is concerned is that they suppress the T cell response and in large doses actually kill lymphocytes outright. Steroids still are a mainstay of treatment for patients with organ transplants, particularly in the early weeks, when the immune response is vigorous and rejection is common. There is, however, an increasing tendency for transplant physicians to try to reduce the dosage of this type of drug as soon as possible (although it usually cannot be wholly discontinued). This is because the long-term administration of steroids in the larger doses necessary to treat repeated episodes of acute cellular rejection can result in a number of complications.

table 6.2

Major Potential Complications of Immunosuppressive Drugs*

Azathioprine

Anemia

Low platelet count (may result in bleeding)

Nausea and vomiting

Diarrhea

Impaired liver function

Skin rashes

Hair loss

Corticosteroids

Peptic ulceration

Pancreatitis

Loss of bone strength (leading to bone fractures)

Collapse of joints

Muscle weakness

Loss of muscle mass

Change in appearance (swollen face and trunk, thin limbs)

Growth retardation in children

Menstrual irregularities in women

Impotence in men

Diabetes

Disturbances of fluid and salt balance

Increased blood levels of cholesterol and triglycerides

Psychiatric complications

Convulsions

Eye disorders (cataracts, glaucoma)

Acne

Spontaneous bleeding into the skin

Disfiguring skin striae (stretch marks)

Antithymocyte globulin

Anaphylactic shock (sudden circulatory collapse)

Muscle and joint pains

Skin rashes

Fever and chills

Asthma attacks

Cyclosporine

Impaired kidney function

Neurological disorders (e.g., tremors)

High blood pressure

Increased blood levels of cholesterol and triglycerides

Increased facial and body hair growth

Thickening of the gums around the teeth

Loss of bone strength

OKT3

Fever and chills

Meningitis

Diarrhea

Tacrolimus

Impaired kidney function

Neurological disorders (e.g., tremors, insomnia, headaches, convulsions, coma)

Diabetes

Increased levels of blood cholesterol and triglycerides

Gastrointestinal disorders (diarrhea)

Hair loss

Mycophenolate mofetil

Nausea and vomiting

Problems with urination

Anemia

Low platelet count (may result in bleeding)

---

*Any and all immunosuppressive drugs, in sufficient dosage or in combination, increase the patient's susceptibility to infection and to malignant tumor formation.

(Table 6.2 is included to provide some idea of the range of these potential complications, but not to unduly worry anyone who is taking a steroid for any medical reason.)

Another drug introduced in the 1960s is of quite a different nature, even though its ultimate effect is similar to azathioprine's. It is known variously as antithymocyte globulin (ATG) or antilymphocyte serum (ALS) and, like azathioprine and steroids, it is still in regular use today. Whereas azathioprine is a drug that is synthesized chemically, ATG is what is known as a biological agent, which in this case means that it is made in an animal. Human T cells are injected into, say, a rabbit, whose immune system recognizes the human cells as foreign and therefore produces antibodies to destroy them. The serum of the rabbit, which contains the antibodies, is then collected and injected into a patient who is rejecting a transplanted organ. The rabbit antihuman-T-cell antibodies destroy the human T cells that are invading the transplanted organ, and the rejection episode is prevented or reversed. We have therefore in a sense copied nature, which produces its own antibodies to destroy a transplanted pig organ, by using antibodies to destroy cells—in this case human T lymphocytes. Several scientists were involved in the early efforts to develop ATG for use in the treatment of rejection, but among the leaders were another pioneer British transplant surgeon Sir Michael Woodruff, and Harvard surgeons Anthony Monaco and Paul Russell.

These three drugs—azathioprine, steroids, and ATG—saw us through the first 25 years or so of organ transplantation, but often they were less than ideally effective. It was in the late 1970s that a major breakthrough took place. A Swiss immunologist, Jean Borel, working for the pharmaceutical company Sandoz in Basel (now merged with Ciba-Geigy to form Novartis), discovered the amazing properties of a naturally occurring fungus that inhibits the function of T cells rather than killing them. Once again, it was Sir Roy Calne, together with Cambridge transplant immunologist David White, who was responsible for much of the experimental work using this new drug, cyclosporine, and for introducing it successfully into the treatment of organ transplant patients. The results of organ transplantation greatly improved, and organs that had hitherto been impossible or exceedingly difficult to transplant successfully, such as the liver, lung, and pancreas, were able to be transplanted on a regular basis.

A second biological agent, OKT3, produced in mice, functions like ATG in that it also kills T lymphocytes, but it is more specific in its target. Its introduction into clinical practice was by the Massachusetts General Hospital transplant team headed by surgeon Ben Cosimi.

The addition of cyclosporine and OKT3 helped markedly improve the results of organ transplantation and led to immense growth in the number of transplants performed in the Western world. Since the late 1980s and early 1990s, two more important drugs have been added to our armamentarium. Tacrolimus (identified in Japan, and developed largely by the work of Pittsburgh transplant surgeon Tom Starzl) is competing with cyclosporine as the major immunosuppressive agent available to us, and mycophenolate mofetil is beginning to replace azathioprine, raising the total number of effective agents to seven.

New drugs

Of the handful of new drugs currently being tested for their effect on rejection, some are quite different from those previously developed. They do not directly kill or inhibit the T cells, but prevent their activation by blocking an auxiliary mechanism known as costimulation. While these have been shown to have a potent effect in suppressing rejection in experimental animals, there is more to the development of a successful drug than demonstrating its efficacy. Is it safe to use, or does it have dangerous side effects? Is it toxic in the dosage required to prevent or treat rejection? In other words, will it poison the patient before it prevents rejection? And of equal importance in the commercial reality of today's world, where development of a single new drug may cost several hundreds of millions of dollars, is the drug so superior to its existing competitors to warrant this vast expenditure? Those agents that block co-stimulation look impressive. Current data suggest that they will play a major role in the treatment of organ transplant recipients in the future.

Some of the new drugs are of interest to potential xenotransplanters because they not only kill or suppress the T cells that generate the cellular response to an organ graft, but also kill or suppress the B cells that produce the antibodies that are the culprits in antibody-mediated rejection. The hope is that one or more will prove of value in this respect.

One point we must remember, however, is that all immunosuppressive drugs have side effects detrimental to the patient who is taking them. Indeed, it is sometimes said that in organ transplantation, the disease causing organ failure has simply been replaced by another disease, namely, the complications associated with prolonged immunosuppressive therapy.

A brief digression on the topic of immunosuppressive drugs: cyclosporine, tacrolimus, and mycophenolate mofetil, as well as several of the drugs currently under investigation, have been isolated from natural organisms, such as fungi, and there are probably many more valuable agents from such sources that await our discovery. One can almost believe that all of the solutions to our medical ills are hidden somewhere in our beautiful world. Sadly, the more we destroy our natural environment, the less solutions will remain to be found.

Overcoming the Fourth and Final Barrier:
Preventing Chronic Rejection ○ ○ ○

There is one final form of rejection that occurs in allografts and is very likely to occur in xenografts. This is chronic rejection. Unlike other forms of rejection, which can destroy an allograft in minutes, days, or weeks, chronic rejection may take months or years to have any effect whatsoever. It has different effects in different organs. For example, in the heart, it leads to thickening of the arteries very similar to coronary artery disease. In the lung, it may cause narrowing of the airways, leading to increasing difficulty in breathing. In the kidney, it may cause gradual destruction of the glomeruli, where the exchange of substances takes place between the blood and the urine. A rough estimate is that chronic rejection accounts for the failure of approximately 5% of all existing organ transplants each year. This is an estimated 5,000 graft losses annually in the United States alone. Some of these patients go back on the waiting list for a second transplant, thus adding to the already overwhelming problem of supply and demand.

At present, there is no effective treatment for chronic rejection. If it becomes advanced enough, the transplanted organ will steadily fail. In the transplanted heart, for example, the arteries become blocked, the patient undergoes one or more heart attacks (which usually occur without pain, as the transplanted heart has no nerve supply), and the only option, apart from drugs to support the failing heart, is to offer the patient a second transplant.

Chronic rejection is almost certain to occur in transplanted pig organs, even if we can overcome the earlier rejection hurdles. In view of the great difference in tissue type between pig and human, it will probably develop faster than in a human organ. A second transplant may have to be offered to the patient earlier than would be the case with a human organ. Whereas some surgeons are reluctant to offer retransplantation to patients today, in view of the shortage of human organs, the ready availability of a limitless supply of animal organs would greatly reduce this ethical dilemma. Although a second, third, or fourth organ transplant is not ideal, they may well be essential if the patient is to see life through for a few more years, and in this case it will be a huge advantage to have no limit to the supply of donor organs.

An analogy with patients who have undergone replacement of a defective heart valve is apt. Replacement can be with a mechanical or a biological valve.

Mechanical valves can fail for one reason or another, and biological valves (often pig heart valves) tend to degenerate with time. Thousands of patients with mechanical or biological heart valves, who remain active and productive members of society, have therefore had to undergo repeated surgical replacement of the valve. It may be that future groups of patients will have to become accustomed to sequential organ transplants. This is certainly not what most of us would choose for our future, but it is an option that many would choose if death were the only alternative.

Happily, however, some of the drugs currently being investigated may help prevent not only early antibody-mediated rejection but also chronic rejection. It is odd to think that a single drug might help prevent both the most rapid form of rejection and the slowest. Yet, if both are proved to be the result of antibody action, as seems possible, then it is conceivable that a single drug—perhaps one we currently use, perhaps one that will emerge with continued research—will be effective in both cases.

chapter 7

The ''Humanized'' Pig

Manipulating the genes of the donor

Making a Better Pig o o o

To date, in order to successfully transplant human organs, we have had to concentrate our entire effort on modifying the immune system of the patient. When an organ becomes available, as is the case with organs from brain-dead human donors, we have only a few hours before it has to be transplanted. There is no time for us to manipulate the donor's antigens even if this were ethically acceptable. We can only manipulate—indeed, suppress—the rejection response of the potential recipient. Xenotransplantation gives us the first real opportunity to modify the donor organ itself. The more we can do to make the donor organ acceptable to the recipient, therefore, the less we will have to do to suppress the recipient's immune response.

Genetic Engineering: Giving the Pig Human Genes o o o

Genetic engineering, the techniques by which genetic material can be altered so as to change the hereditary properties of an organism or cell, was scientifically impossible when both of the writers of this book were medical students, not that many years ago. Today it is becoming commonplace not only in the laboratory but in actual veterinary practice. For example, genetic engineering is being used to increase milk production in cows and to produce human proteins in goat and cow milk that can be used in the treatment of patients. Together with new cloning technologies and gene therapy, genetic engineering is certain to play an increasingly important role in medical science, particularly in the correction of inherited human conditions.

Laboratory mice can now be engineered in myriad ways for the purposes of exploring normal (or abnormal) body functions. For example, we can investigate the role of certain immune cells, or the products of these cells, in the rejection response. Mice can be engineered so that their immune response is in some way either deficient or excessive, allowing immunologists to investigate normal and abnormal functions as never before. Tremendous amounts of data are being generated, resulting in greatly enhanced understanding of how animals, including humans, function, particularly in relation to the immune system. In mice, this technology has advanced rapidly. A new gene (or genes) can be introduced with relative ease, and in some strains it is possible to delete, or "knock out," an existing gene. In the pig, however, it requires an enormous investment of time and resources if it is to be successful. It is possible to introduce a gene in pigs, but not yet to knock out an existing one. The new gene that is introduced by these genetic engineering techniques is known as a transgene. How are these transgenic animals produced? The following description owes much to expert information provided by Lindsay Williams and his colleagues at Stem Cell Sciences in Melbourne, Australia, a leading biotechnology company in this field.

One first has to accept that the present techniques are extremely inefficient. To have even a modest chance of success, a large number of pigs is required. For example, if 100 embryos (developing piglets) are injected with the required genetic material, then approximately 10 piglets will be born. However, only one or two of these animals are likely to be transgenic, that is, to have incorporated the required genetic material in the right place. Furthermore, the gene may not be expressed as strongly as needed for the intended purpose. This gives an idea of the amount of work that is required to produce even one transgenic animal.

The initial step is to treat the sow with certain hormones (Figure 7.1). This induces superovulation (the production of a large number of eggs). Approximately one day later, the sow is mated with a boar. Within 24 hours, the fertilized eggs (now technically embryos) are retrieved from the sow under anesthesia.

The next step is to inject the foreign genetic material—the transgene DNA—into the embryos using microscopic techniques. (Figure 7.2). The hope is that these foreign genes will be incorporated into the cell's genetic repertoire. This requires considerable skill and the use of pipettes or needles no thicker than the diameter of a human hair. The disadvantage of this technique is that the foreign DNA is randomly integrated into the embryo's chro-

figure 7.1. *Major steps in creating a transgenic animal.*

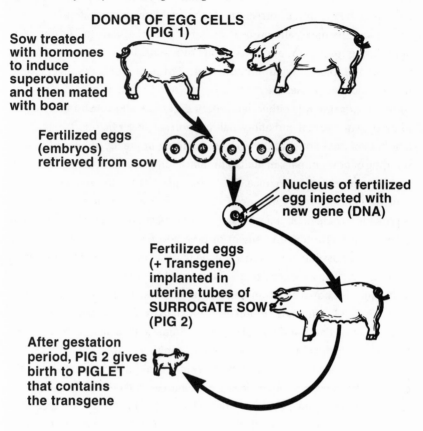

DONOR OF EGG CELLS
(PIG 1)

Sow treated
with hormones
to induce
superovulation
and then mated
with boar

Fertilized eggs
(embryos)
retrieved from sow

Nucleus of fertilized
egg injected with
new gene (DNA)

Fertilized eggs
(+ Transgene)
implanted in
uterine tubes of
SURROGATE SOW
(PIG 2)

After gestation
period, PIG 2 gives
birth to PIGLET
that contains
the transgene

mosomes; in other words, there is no control over where the new DNA will end up in the chromosomes, or how many copies of the gene will become part of the recipient cell.

The embryos are then implanted into the uterus of surrogate sows that have been superovulated and mated with a sterile boar. Approximately 25 embryos are introduced into each sow. The pregnancy is then allowed to progress to term. Only about 10% of these embryos will go on to develop as piglets. Each piglet must then be tested to ascertain whether the desired gene is expressed in its cells; usually this has been achieved in only between 10 and 20%. In other words, only perhaps 1 of the original 25 injected embryos may have developed into a transgenic piglet, but even this piglet may not express the gene well.

When a successful transgenic piglet is born, the next step is to breed from it. Both male and female transgenic pigs can transmit the gene to their

figure 7.2. *Microinjection of a transgene into a pig egg, performed under the microscope. The diameter of the egg is approximately 70 microns (micrometers, μm; 1 micron = 0.001 mm). The holding pipette used (to the left) is between 15 and 50 microns in diameter, whereas the injection pipette (to the right) is approximately 0.75 micron in diameter. (Courtesy of Stem Cell Sciences, Melbourne, Australia.)*

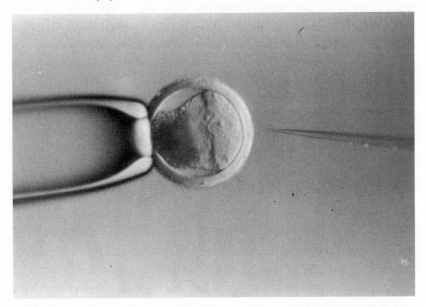

offspring, but it is advantageous to use transgenic boars whenever possible, as these can quickly inseminate many different sows. A sow becomes capable of bearing piglets at the age of about six months and is ready to be mated every three weeks. Pregnancy takes between 112 to 117 days, and so it is about 9–12 months before a newborn piglet can deliver its own offspring. Although commercial sows may give birth to a litter of 8–12 young, more highly inbred sows may have fewer than half this number of offspring. The time it takes, therefore, to produce a relatively large herd of transgenic pigs is not inconsiderable. The costs associated with this enterprise are, of course, significant.

Development of a Gal-negative pig

Let us now return to the problem of modifying a donor pig to protect its organs from hyperacute rejection. Approaches to modifying the donor organ are concentrated in two key areas—the antibody-antigen binding that takes place after the organ is transplanted into a human recipient, and the subsequent complement-induced destruction that occurs.

It would clearly be advantageous to remove or change the expression of the important Gal sugar on the lining of the pig blood vessels. If Gal could be removed, replaced, or masked, there would be no target for human anti-pig antibodies, and therefore no activation of the complement cascade. In practice, however, it is not proving that simple. Studies in mice suggest that there may be other targets "hidden" under the Gal epitope. Nevertheless, if we could prevent the expression of the Gal sugar on the blood vessels, the single most important target for human anti-pig antibodies would no longer be a factor in the conundrum we are trying to solve. To use an image from chess, it would be equivalent to capturing the opponent's queen.

"Gal knockout": knocking out the sugar

The first approach was suggested a few years ago both by our group in Oklahoma City and independently by two groups of scientists in Melbourne, Australia, at St. Vincent's Hospital and the Austin Research Institute. The idea was to genetically engineer a pig that simply did not produce the Gal sugar. The technology necessary to do this—the so-called gene knockout technique—is available in the mouse but unfortunately not yet in the pig. The reason for this is that the technique is dependent on obtaining stem cells from the animal. Stem cells are very primitive unspecialized cells that are the precursors of other, more differentiated cells. That is, they have the ability to develop into cells with any of a number of functions, such as nerve, skin, or muscle cells. In other words, they remain pluripotent. While stem cells cannot yet be identified in the pig and removed for subsequent manipulation, it is nevertheless interesting to explore how Gal could potentially be deleted.

The Gal sugar in the pig is produced by an enzyme called α-1, 3-galactosyltransferase—GT for short. This enzyme has the job of attaching a Gal molecule to an underlying (substrate) sugar—in this case to a basic lactosamine sugar. GT is encoded by a single gene, which directs the production of the enzyme. If this single gene could be knocked out, then the GT enzyme that adds the Gal sugar would be eliminated. Theoretically, at least, this would be ideal, as such a modified pig would be born with no Gal targets for human anti-pig antibodies to attack (Figure 7.3).

Humans, apes, and Old World monkeys actually have a primitive non-functioning gene which cannot make the GT enzyme. This is why these species do not produce the problematic sugar. Since these species live perfectly well without any Gal, as do mice that have had the Gal-expressing gene removed, there seems no reason to believe that knockout (Gal-negative) pigs would not thrive equally successfully.

figure 7.3. *Strategies to disrupt the synthesis of the Gal sugar by genetic engineering techniques in the pig. Ideally, the α-1, 3-galactosyltransferase (GT) gene could be "knocked out" (top), but this is not yet technically possible in the pig. A GT knockout pig would express no Gal. Gal can be partially eliminated by the enzyme α-galactosidase, which removes terminal Gal sugar molecules (left). An alternative transgenic approach is to insert the gene for the enzyme α-1, 2-fucosyltransferase (FT) which competes with the GT for utilization of the substrate (lactosamine) and forms the branched O blood group sugar (right). This partially eliminates production of Gal. The insertion of both FT and galactosidase genes may result in a pig that expresses no Gal (bottom).*

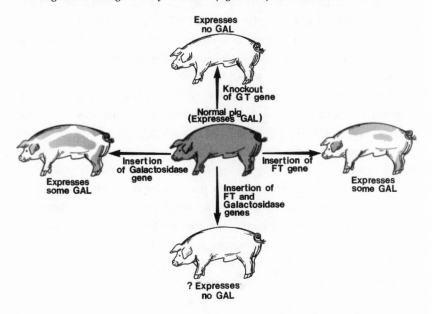

Gal-knockout mice

Although this technology is not yet available in the pig, strains of Gal-knockout (that is, Gal-negative) mice have been successfully bred in at least two laboratories, one in Australia and one in the United States. In the absence of Gal, the other sugars that are present on the lining of the blood vessels—sialic acid and lactosamine, and possibly others—take over the space vacated by the Gal. However, work predominantly from the laboratory of immunologist Tony d'Apice at St. Vincent's Hospital in Melbourne has demonstrated that these Gal-negative mouse organs are still susceptible to damage caused by human serum. The reason for this remains uncertain; it may be that once the Gal is removed from the blood vessels, newly exposed sugars (the nature of which remains uncertain at present) are recognized by other (non-anti-Gal) human antibodies. Although the speed of rejection is diminished, human antibodies still cause damage to the mouse organ. Whatever the mechanism, the bottom line unfortunately is that the absence of Gal does not protect the donor organ as completely as had been anticipated.

One interesting observation made in these Gal-deficient mice is that in the absence of any Gal in their bodies, they soon develop antibodies directed against this sugar. Just as the newborn human infant produces anti-Gal antibodies when its gut is colonized by Gal-expressing bacteria, so these Gal-deficient mice do the same. This strain of mouse is therefore proving extremely useful as an inexpensive model for investigating these antibodies further, as the animals can serve as a surrogate for the human or baboon in this regard. Indeed, though they have not provided us with the whole answer we were hoping for, they are greatly facilitating research in this field.

Transplantation of a normal mouse heart (one that expresses Gal) into a Gal-negative knockout mouse that produces anti-Gal antibodies, however, does not fully mimic the pig-to-baboon transplant model. Although we are testing the same antigen-antibody system, we are dealing with mouse-to-mouse allografts and not with xenografts. Both donor and recipient mice have the same complement regulatory proteins on their cell surfaces. Furthermore, except for Gal, all of the other antigens on the cell surfaces are either identical or extremely similar between the two strains of mouse (Gal-knockout and wild-type). The mouse model, although helpful to us, is therefore not a true reflection of the problems we face in pig-to-primate xenotransplantation.

Competing with Gal

Although an existing gene cannot yet be deleted in a pig, a new gene can be successfully introduced by the DNA injection technique outlined at the beginning of this chapter. An alternative to the Gal-knockout pig was therefore suggested by the Oklahoma City and Austin Research Institute groups. The strategy is to breed a pig that expresses another carbohydrate structure that competes with, and with luck replaces, the Gal sugar on the blood vessel lining. For example, a pig could be genetically engineered to carry the sugar found in people with type O blood. Since the vast majority of humans do not have antibodies to this sugar, the pig organ would not elicit an antibody-mediated response when transplanted into a patient.

The possibility of modifying pig tissue in this way has been termed "competitive glycosylation" (when two or more sugars compete for attachment to the same site). In the normal pig, the sugar lactosamine is utilized as the substrate in the production of the Gal sugar. The enzyme GT attaches a Gal terminal sugar onto the lactosamine. The O blood group sugar also uses lac-

figure 7.4. *Organs from pigs genetically engineered to carry branched sugar groups on their blood vessels (found in people with type O blood) should be protected from human-antibody-mediated rejection. The human anti-Gal antibodies can no longer bind to the sugar chains lining the pig blood vessels, and therefore complement is not activated. (Compare with Figure 5.2, p. 63.)*

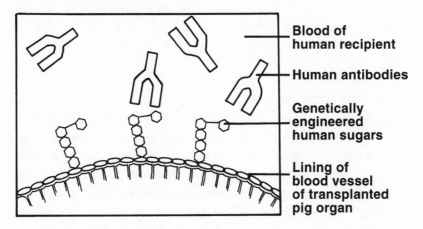

Blood of human recipient

Human antibodies

Genetically engineered human sugars

Lining of blood vessel of transplanted pig organ

tosamine as its base but, in this case, the α-1, 2-fucosyltransferase enzyme (FT, for short) adds a molecule that differs in structure from Gal (see Figure 7.4, and compare it with Figure 5.2). If the gene for FT is introduced into the pig, the enzyme should compete with GT for the available lactosamine substrate.

Experiments have been carried out in cell culture and in transgenic mice (and, recently, in a very small number of transgenic pigs). When the gene for FT has been introduced, the enzyme does indeed compete successfully with GT for the lactosamine substrate; about 90% of the lactosamine is covered with the O sugar, leaving only 10% covered with Gal (see Figure 7.3). Mauro Sandrin, Ian McKenzie, and their colleagues at Melbourne's Austin Research Institute have discovered that FT competes so successfully with GT because FT appears to function earlier than GT in what is known as the Golgi apparatus of the cell and thus has "first choice" of the available lactosamine. Once again, however, Tony d'Apice's group has demonstrated that the rearrangement in the sugar distribution on the surface of the blood vessels could be detrimental because it may potentially expose other (unknown) sugar antigens, which could be targets for antibodies, although the Austin group has not observed significant changes in this respect.

Uri Galili has estimated that, depending on the type of cell, there are between 10 million and 30 million Gal molecules exposed on the surface of every pig cell. (This works out to 1 trillion Gal molecules in every gram of the cells lining the pig's blood vessels.) Unfortunately, the number is so great that replacing even 90% of them will not be sufficient to prevent hyperacute rejection of a pig organ transplanted into a patient, as the remaining 1 million to 3 million Gal molecules will certainly provide enough sites for the anti-Gal antibodies to destroy the organ. We therefore have to find some way to eliminate the remaining Gal molecules. One strategy might be to combine manipulations, perhaps introducing not one but two new genes into the pig cells.

Two are better than one

Just as there is an enzyme that manufactures and attaches Gal sugar molecules, there is another enzyme, α-galactosidase—that *removes* this sugar, cleaving Gal from, rather than attaching it to, the lactosamine base. While the idea might seem promising, in practice the results have been frustrating. The galactosidase enzyme does not remove all of the Gal terminal molecules, leaving between 30 and 40% undisturbed. Perhaps some of these sugars are not removable because they are in deep "crevices" on the cell membrane; far from being smooth, a cell membrane is in fact a very irregular surface, with long chains of glycoproteins (sugars connected to proteins) sticking out and interspersed with shorter chains of glycolipids (sugars connected to fats).

Despite these frustrations, the puzzle may yet be resolved, thanks in large part to the work of Mauro Sandrin, Ian McKenzie, and their colleagues. Although their work is only in the cell culture stage, they have shown that when both the gene for FT and that for galactosidase are inserted into a cell that produces the Gal sugar, 100% of the Gal is replaced (see Figure 7.3). The FT replaces 90% of the Gal sugar with the human O blood group sugar, and the galactosidase removes the Gal molecules that remain after the FT has done its initial work. This may enable the underlying lactosamine substrate to be "recycled"—to be made available to the FT for a second try, so to speak. The FT obliges by attaching more of the O sugar, thus completing the replacement of Gal. This exciting work is only now progressing into mice, and is some way from reaching the point of a trial in pigs, but the results to date have been encouraging.

We may ultimately end up with a pig that expresses the universal donor O sugar rather than Gal—at least that's the theory. But as in most areas of biological research, the solution may not be as simple as we hope. Nature has a habit of placing unexpected hurdles in our way. For example, pigs have their own FT gene and produce the O sugar without any help from us. This sugar is present in many tissues of the pig's body, but for complex reasons is *not* present on the lining of the blood vessels, which for us is the crucial structure, inasmuch as the blood vessels are the first structure with which human anti-pig antibodies will come into contact. It is essential, therefore, that we "persuade" the pig—via our transgenic technology—to express the O sugar on these essential cells. This could conceivably prove a stumbling block, for why does the pig's gene for the FT enzyme not express the O sugar on the blood vessel lining?

The first attempt to breed a pig that expresses the O sugar on its blood vessels was carried out in the laboratory of surgeon Hiroshi Takagi in Nagoya, Japan. The resulting pig rapidly developed multiple tumors in its bowel, and died within a few months. Such malignancies are extremely rare in young pigs. Although this observation is very preliminary, it may be that a radical change in the sugar pattern somehow predisposes pigs to tumor formation. With advances in the technology, the reasons for this may be identified, and perhaps subsequent attempts may have a different outcome.

Protection against human complement

The other major approach involving the use of genetic engineering to prevent hyperacute rejection is to leave the Gal sugars intact and concentrate on preventing the complement-induced injury. Nature has arranged it so that animals are protected against complement of their own species. This species-specificity of complement and its regulatory proteins suggested to ingenious scientists—such as Augustin Dalmasso of Minneapolis, Minnesota, and David White of Cambridge, United Kingdom—a potential method of protecting pig organs from human complement. They suggested that a gene responsible for the production of one of the human complement-regulatory proteins—there are several—should be transferred into pigs. These pigs would now express not only pig complement-regulatory proteins but also one of the human complement-regulatory proteins. The resulting pig would be protected, at least to some extent, from injury by both pig and human complement.

A number of groups in the United Kingdom, United States, and Australia are developing this technology, using the genes for several different complement-regulatory proteins. The most common proteins investigated to date are known as decay accelerating factor (abbreviated to DAF), membrane cofactor protein (MCP), and membrane inhibitor of reactive lysis (CD59). DAF has proven particularly successful in protecting pig cells. This technology has been advanced primarily by a group headed by immunologist David White at the University of Cambridge and the U.K. biotechnology company Imutran.

Organs from pigs transgenically manipulated to express human DAF have been transplanted into monkeys and baboons. These xenografts have proved almost universally resistant to the hyperacute rejection caused by complement injury, although this protection extends only for a few days and eventually either anti-pig antibodies overwhelm the capacity of the human DAF to protect the transplanted organ or delayed destruction takes place by other ill-defined mechanisms, which may be independent of complement. When the recipient monkeys were given heavy immunosuppressive drug therapy, which at least partially suppressed antibody production and possibly some of these other mechanisms, some of the transplanted pig organs continued to function for longer than one or even two months. However, the heavy doses of immunosuppressants were associated with considerable toxicity. Some experiments had to be terminated on humane grounds because of the development of health problems, such as diarrhea and weight loss, in the monkeys. Nevertheless, this experience is certainly an extremely encouraging beginning to the use of genetic engineering in xenotransplantation. Of all the strategies to prevent hyperacute rejection and extend pig organ survival that have been discussed in this volume, the use of organs from such transgenic pigs has proved the most successful to date.

These experiments suggest that, as with CVF and sCR1, pig organs protected from injury from human complement alone will prove insufficient and further modifications of the donor pig and/or recipient human will be required. With experience and further advances in genetic engineering, however, greater expression of human complement-regulatory proteins on pig organs is likely to be achieved. The expression of two or more complement-regulatory proteins may confer greater protection than one alone. Indeed, Tony d'Apice's group and others have already demonstrated this in mice. It would also seem likely that a pig transgenic for human DAF but also for FT and galactosidase might provide added protection. The possibilities are numerous and will continue to be explored by several groups during the next few years.

These initial observations from Cambridge—more recently supported by work from the Princeton-based biotechnology company Nextran—also suggest that despite efforts to modify the donor organ, immunosuppressive drug therapy may be required at such massive doses that it will prove unfeasible in humans. It may be that long-term survival of pig organs in humans will only be achieved if the recipient can be rendered "tolerant" to the transplanted organ, as will be discussed in the next chapter. There is, however, another technology that has received much recent publicity, cloning, and this might well facilitate the genetic modification of the donor organ.

Cloning, the Newest Technology o o o

Unlike in a transgenic animal, where only a gene or a small fragment of DNA is introduced into the host cell, in cloning the entire genetic template of an animal is introduced into the shell of an egg cell. Cloning therefore opens up a number of exciting possibilities for xenotransplantation. These extend from cloning individual cells and tissues for the treatment of disorders such as diabetes or Parkinson's disease to the economic production of large numbers of pigs bearing the genetic traits necessary to resist rejection by the human immune system.

Keith Campbell of the Scottish biotechnology company PPL Therapeutics—which, with the associated Roslin Institute, is a leader in this field—has described cloning (also called nuclear transfer) as "the reconstruction of an embryo by the transfer of genetic material from a single donor cell to an unfertilized egg from which the genetic material has been removed." Campbell points out that the resultant offspring will not actually be true clones, as they will inherit some components of the maternal egg that are in the cytoplasm and not part of the nucleus (e.g., mitochondria, which have their own genetic system). There will therefore be subtle differences between offspring and the genetic donor of the nuclear material. However, for practical purposes the offspring can be considered as genomic copies of the donor of the nuclear material.

In cloning, a single cell is stimulated to divide, multiply, and differentiate into all of the multitude of specialized cells that make up an adult animal. It is easy to make a cell multiply, but the nature of the cells generally remains the same as that of the initial cell. For example, fibroblasts, which produce collagen, one of the key structural elements of the body, multiply to produce more fibroblasts. The breakthrough that has taken place has been the ability to coax what is called a terminally differentiated cell, such as a fibroblast, to divide into the many other types of cell—brain, muscle, intestinal, and so on—that make up a fully formed animal. It was previously believed that once a cell had differentiated into its specialized form, it could not be induced or manipulated to develop into any other forms of specialized cell, but the work reported from the Roslin Institute–PPL Therapeutics group in Scotland in 1997 demonstrates this fundamental perception is wrong.

Although the cloning of the sheep named Dolly (Figure 7.5)—the first mammal cloned from a single adult cell—captured the world's attention in 1997, the cloning of animals from immature cells (cells that have not already differentiated into specialized cells, but still retain an ability to do this) had been reported previously. As far back as the 1950s, pioneering biologists—

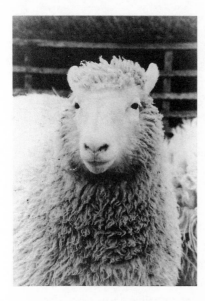

figure 7.5. *Dolly, the first mammal to be cloned from an adult cell.*

most notably Sir John Gurdon, then at Oxford University and now at Cambridge—had started to perfect the critical technique of nuclear transfer. Cloned tadpoles and even adult frogs were successfully raised using this approach. But this could only be achieved when the cells used for the nuclear transfer procedure were very immature—embryonic or fetal cells. The older the donor cell, the less likely the clone was to develop normally. For example, when nuclei from adult frog cells were used in these experiments, none of the frog clones ever developed beyond the juvenile tadpole stage. The larvae developed eyes and external gills, but halfway through their metamorphosis to adulthood, they died. The results were even more discouraging in mice, one of the simplest mammalian models.

Researchers at the Roslin Institute suggested that these failures were not caused by some irreversible process that occurs during differentiation (the changes that turn embryonic cells into specialized muscle, nerves, and other body tissues) but rather were the result of the cloning procedure itself. Using technical modifications of their own and the nuclear transfer technique (Figure 7.6), they first cloned fully formed, normal sheep from embryo-derived differentiated cells, and in 1996 reported the birth of two healthy lambs, Megan and Morag. They then went on to extend this success by cloning sheep from fetal fibroblasts (cells that had already matured from the embryonic state but were still relatively immature) and finally by creating a sheep, Dolly, from a single cell from an adult ewe's udder.

figure 7.6. *Major steps in the technique of nuclear transfer (cloning). Although cloning of a pig is illustrated in this figure, the technique of nuclear transfer is difficult in this species and has been successful only using very early embryonic cells. It has been more successful with sheep, goats, cattle, and mice. The donor of the nuclear material (pig 1) is usually an embryo or fetus rather than an adult pig.*

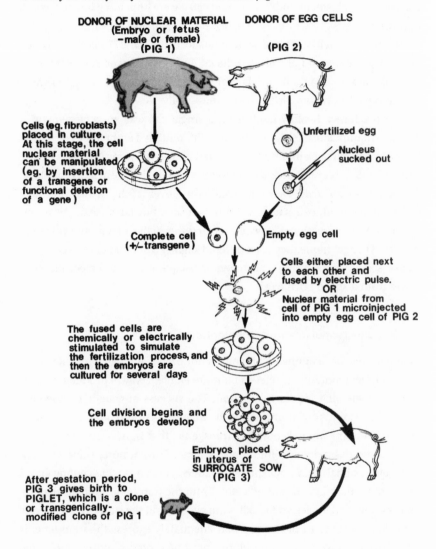

In Dolly's case, the udder cells were fused with unfertilized sheep eggs whose own chromosomes had been removed—only the surrounding cytoplasm and cellular machinery necessary to allow the cell to develop remained. About a week later, the resulting embryos (which at this stage consisted of a cluster of undifferentiated cells) were implanted into the womb of surrogate ewes. However, even using their ingenious innovations, this procedure proved inefficient and largely unsuccessful. Of 277 eggs into which the new genetic material was introduced, only 29 embryos survived longer than six days and could be implanted into surrogate ewes, and all of these 29 embryos died before birth, except one—Dolly.

To produce a healthy lamb from a single cell was an achievement in itself. To manipulate a relatively mature, differentiated embryonic cell so that it could be taken back in time and reverted to its embryonic state was clearly a remarkable achievement and constitutes a major advance in biotechnology. To then go on to wield the same magic wand over a fully mature and fully differentiated adult cell is a truly significant scientific advance. In 1998, scientists at the University of Hawaii repeated this achievement, but this time in mice. The technique they used differed slightly from that employed by the British scientists. Japanese researchers subsequently cloned eight identical calves from a single bovine cell.

Cloning's potential in xenotransplantation

Although this new cloning technology is not practical on a large scale at the present time, it potentially offers a far more efficient way of producing transgenic animals for xenotransplantation. The success of genetic engineering techniques is not known until after the offspring is born, and only a small proportion of the animals born are transgenic, that is, have successfully integrated the desired genes into their genome. Furthermore, some of these transgenic animals may not express the added gene(s) at a high enough level to be functionally effective or efficient. From the transgenic animals that are successfully bred, males and females are chosen and the slow process begins of raising a large herd of animals that adequately express the transgene. It may therefore take years to develop a herd of several hundred transgenic sheep or pigs.

In contrast, Dolly-style cloning can be used to immediately churn out as many identical copies of a transgenic animal as needed *in a single generation*. The cell is modified as required and then multiple copies of the modified cell are used to breed an almost instantaneous flock or herd. Although the currently available techniques do not obviate the randomness and trial and error of transgenesis, the success or failure of the manipulations can be assessed early at the cellular level rather than proceeding with the costly and wasteful process of breeding a large number of animals. For xenotransplantation, the gene of interest—for example, that for FT or human DAF, or both—could be inserted into the nuclear material of the cell. The desired cell would be multiplied many times, and these cells fused individually with the cytoplasmic shells of enucleated eggs. The resulting fused cells would then be placed in surrogate sows. Less than four months later, multiple piglets (possibly hundreds) would be born expressing the desired gene.

In this regard, Dolly's creators have already extended their success by using fetal cells to clone animals that carry a foreign implanted gene. The researchers inserted human genes into the nuclei of fetal fibroblasts to clone three lambs (Polly and two others). The human gene was that for the factor IX protein, which is used to treat patients with a serious disorder of blood clotting, which has the rather interesting name of Christmas disease (or hemophilia B). Such transgenic lambs will produce this human clotting factor in their milk, making them relatively inexpensive and plentiful suppliers of this important therapeutic agent.

Similar results have been achieved in cows using a variation of this technique. A team at Advanced Cell Technology in Massachusetts cloned the first transgenic calves, George and Charlie, carrying a foreign marker gene. In collaboration with Genzyme Transgenics, this company has now created the beginnings of herds of cows and goats that produce in their milk human albumin and various pharmaceutical drugs for use in patients. The births of all of these animals are remarkable, not only because the animals are clones, but because they demonstrate that cloning works even after genetic modification of a cell.

Although not achieved to date, cloning also creates the potential for making absolutely precise genetic changes within a cell by gene targeting, knockout, and substitution. This would allow an unwanted gene, such as the GT gene, to be deleted within the cell, which will then be cloned to produce a herd of animals that do not express the gene. The ability to genetically modify animals in this way will prove a great advantage for the economic production of humanized animal organ and tissue donors.

There has already been work that demonstrates that nuclear transfer can be successful in mice and primates, which suggests that it is feasible in all mammalian species, including the pig. Success in the pig—our chosen animal for xenotransplantation—has not yet been achieved. Pig egg cells are hard to activate and difficult to culture and maintain in the absence of fertilization before their implantation into surrogate sows. At the time of writing,

however, recent progress suggests that successful cloning of a pig is immi-
nent.

Cloning and tissue transplants

Faced with the reality of successful cloning, biologists are now considering
harnessing the nuclear transfer technique to clone individual cells as opposed to whole animals. It might eventually prove possible, for example, to
obtain a specific differentiated cell from an animal, perhaps modify this cell
genetically to resist rejection or to produce greater amounts of a therapeutic
substance such as insulin, and then transfer the DNA of the cell into an
unfertilized egg from which the DNA has been removed. Cultivated in the
laboratory, these cells would begin to divide. Growth factors would be added
to the culture dishes to stimulate multiplication so that literally millions of
the desired cell type would be produced. In this case, the cells would be
positively discouraged from differentiating into a whole animal. They would
not be implanted into a surrogate mother or allowed to differentiate into an
embryo. The aim would be only to clone identical cells for various human
disorders, such as islets for diabetics, or new skin for burn victims, or even
retinal tissue for patients at risk of blindness. Cloned transgenic bovine neurons have already been used experimentally to treat the degenerative disorder
of Parkinson's disease in rats.

Of course, if this can be achieved with animal cells, it should also be
possible with a human patient's own cells. This might enable large numbers
of human tissue transplants to be carried out rather than face the immunological problems associated with xenografting. A burned patient's own skin
cells could be cloned, providing him with grafts that would not be rejected.
The possibilities are enormous, but the science—and the ethics—is in its
infancy. For example, the potential of cloning a human individual to supply
spare body parts for transplantation has given rise to much concern and a
call for legislation to ban human reproductive cloning. Cloning's ultimate
role in both allotransplantation and xenotransplantation remains to be seen.

chapter 8

The Immunological Holy Grail

Tolerance

The Limitations of Present-Day
Immunosuppressive Drugs ○ ○ ○

His heart transplant was necessary because he had suffered three heart attacks during the past eight years. He initially did well; he was out of the
hospital within three weeks and experienced only one early rejection episode.
This was treated successfully, and he returned to work as a business executive
within three months. Six weeks later a viral pneumonia put him back in the
intensive care unit. He recovered from this within a month, only to relapse
with a mild stomach upset from the same virus. Having once again returned
to work, he began to experience low back pain, which he attributed to sitting
at a desk all day long. It troubled him most days, and he had to increase the
painkillers he was taking. His doctors said his bones were getting thin and
prescribed calcium tablets. Still, life was generally very good until he developed cancer of the lymph nodes in his neck four years later. His immunosuppressive drugs were reduced and he underwent a course of radiation
therapy, which seemed to cure him, although the possibility of a recurrence
remained at the back of his mind.

Five years after his transplant, his annual coronary arteriogram indicated
thickening of the arteries in his transplanted heart. Although he was told this
represented chronic rejection, it caused no disability for a further three years.
By that time it had progressed to the point where he was experiencing difficulty in breathing whenever he did even modest exercise such as walking his

dog. His transplanted heart was failing. He discussed retransplantation with his doctors but they didn't seem too keen on this idea in view of his weakened bones, his past history of cancer, and the deteriorating function of his kidneys. He was forced to give up walking the dog and, much more importantly, he had to resign from his job.

Reading, television, and his computer now filled his days. One evening his wife found him dead seated in front of the television. It was just three weeks short of the 10th anniversary of his transplant. At his funeral, his pastor gave thanks for the 10 years of extended life the transplant had given him, but of course the patient and his family would have liked 10 or 20 more.

Despite the success of present-day immunosuppressive drugs, approximately half of all patients with human organ transplants will have lost their grafts (or died) within 10 years from the time of the transplant. The major cause of failure of the transplanted organ after the first year is chronic rejection. Although this develops in almost every patient with time, a small number retain good graft function for 20 or even 30 years. Unfortunately, the currently available drugs do not prevent this late complication. Some of the newer drugs may be more successful, but we shall have to wait for 5 to 10 years to assess their effect.

There is also a small loss of transplant patients over the years from complications such as infection and cancer, both associated with the need to give the patients immunosuppressive drug therapy every day of their lives. Many other less serious problems also result from the side effects of these drugs (see Table 6.2). For example, steroids cause loss of bone strength, particularly of the spine, and some patients suffer complications from this in the form of collapsed vertebrae, leading to backache and sometimes symptoms similar to those of a slipped disc. Cyclosporine and tacrolimus can slowly damage the kidneys. It is the very drugs that have enabled patients to survive through the first few months and years without rejecting their transplanted kidney, heart, or liver that are one of the major causes of late complications.

The Concept of Tolerance ○ ○ ○

It would be wonderful if the patient could accept a graft, either from a human donor or from a pig, without the need for any long-term drug therapy. Such a state, where the body accepts the foreign organ without any form of continuing drug therapy, is known as immunological tolerance. The grafted organ is tolerated by the host as if it were its own, and the patient's body no longer tries to reject it.

This tolerance is donor-specific and would therefore be extended only to the transplanted organ or to other tissues from the same donor. Organs or tissues from any other human donor (unless an identical twin of the first donor) would be rejected in the normal fashion. Following xenografting of an organ from a pig to a human, only tissues from that one donor pig would be tolerated, unless the pig has an identical littermate or had been cloned.

Following both allografting and xenografting, therefore, the immunologically tolerant patient would retain the ability to reject invading bacteria and other microorganisms (or grafted organs from other donors) without impairment. This is clearly more desirable than administering immunosuppressive drugs, which to some extent suppress all aspects of the patient's immune response, including the protective response to infectious organisms. This inevitably puts the patient at risk from certain troublesome, and sometimes life-threatening, infections throughout his or her lifetime.

Furthermore, the induction of tolerance does not impair the ability of the patient's immune system to seek out and destroy cells undergoing malignant (cancerous) change. The risk of developing cancer is very high in patients who have received immunosuppressive drugs for many years, particularly if at times the dosages of these drugs have been heavy and have included the biological agents ATG and OKT3. For example, the risk of a cancer developing in a patient with a human heart transplant is 100 times greater than in the general public. Fortunately, many of these tumors are skin cancers, which can usually be successfully treated by surgical excision or irradiation. Unfortunately, more serious tumors also occur more commonly than in the general population. Many of these are the result of malignant changes developing in the lymphocyte population of white blood cells, leading to tumors known as lymphomas. Since it is possible that even higher doses of immunosuppressive drugs may be required to suppress rejection of a xenografted pig organ, the incidence of cancer in these patients may be even greater. Prevention of this complication would be a major advantage of the induction of tolerance.

Finally, if true tolerance can be achieved, not only will the patient not suffer from early acute rejection episodes, but neither will he or she develop the later chronic rejection that frequently leads to graft failure after several years of good function. There is also preliminary evidence that a state of tolerance can be induced that will prevent hyperacute rejection—the very early rejection of pig xenografts by antibodies.

Much experimental work has been carried out in attempts to achieve tolerance in recipients of organ transplants. To achieve this state, one method is to temporarily deplete or paralyze the patient's immune system while the donor organ is inserted. This requires a much more profound manipulation of the immune system than is achieved by standard immunosuppressive drug therapy. During the period of paralysis, which is only for a few days, the body acclimates to the presence of the transplanted organ and no longer treats it as foreign. When the immune response recovers, the body accepts the organ as its own—as "self" rather than "non-self"—without the need for any immunosuppressive drug therapy. The patient remains fully protected against all invading microorganisms and is able to maintain a normal surveillance against cells undergoing cancerous change.

The ability to successfully transplant animal organs into humans has been one of the holy grails of transplant immunologists and surgeons for many years; immunological tolerance has been the other. In fact, until recently, the search for a means of inducing tolerance to an allograft has been a more urgent quest than that for a means of enabling animal organs to be used. Researchers attempting to achieve tolerance to pig organs—among whose number is one of the authors of this volume—have therefore set themselves a difficult task: they are seeking both holy grails at one time.

In Search of Tolerance o o o

The South African experience

In the world of organ transplantation, South Africa is best known for the pioneering work of Cape Town heart surgeon Christiaan Barnard, who gained enormous public recognition in the late 1960s. The number of medical centers in that country involved in transplantation research during the past 30 to 40 years has been small, and, with the present government's priority on improving basic health care for a greater proportion of the population, this number is certain to fall even further. Nevertheless, South African surgeons have made some significant contributions in this field.

In the late 1970s and early 1980s, pioneering work on immunological tolerance was carried out in Johannesburg. Transplant surgeon Johannes (Bertie) Myburgh and his team at the University of the Witwatersrand achieved this state (or something closely approximating it) in baboons that received kidney transplants from unrelated baboons. The recipient baboon was given a course of radiation directed mainly at the thymus and lymph glands that harbor and regulate the T lymphocytes in the body (so-called total lymphoid irradiation). While the immune system was profoundly but temporarily suppressed by this therapy, the donor organ was inserted. When the host's immune system recovered (which could take from a few days to weeks), it had lost its memory and had to re-educate itself about which tissues it should protect (its own) and which it should destroy (foreign invaders). Every cell and organ present in the body *at that time* were considered to be "self" rather than foreign. The newly developing immune cells had thus been tricked into accepting the kidney as its own, and so did not attempt to destroy it.

This form of therapy was then attempted in a number of patients undergoing kidney transplants in Johannesburg. Unfortunately, the results were not as successful as in the experimental laboratory. One of the main reasons for this was that in the hospital it was not possible to time the kidney transplant to coincide exactly with the radiation therapy used to induce the state of tolerance. By contrast, in the laboratory both the recipient and donor baboons could be selected ahead of time. Although the prospective recipient, the patient, could be identified, the surgeons had no idea when a suitable human donor kidney would become available. The patient would therefore undergo the therapy to allow a donor organ to be transplanted but, if no donor became available at that time, the optimum time would pass and the immune system would recover. Booster doses of irradiation were given at intervals in an attempt to keep the patient in the ideal state to accept the transplanted kidney, but it was unfortunately rarely possible to transplant a kidney when the patient's immune system was fully suppressed and receptive to tolerate the donor organ. The kidney was therefore generally transplanted at a suboptimal time. Nevertheless, although full tolerance was not achieved, these patients required less immunosuppressive drug therapy than most kidney transplant patients. This was clearly of benefit in reducing the incidence of the drug-related complications outlined earlier in this chapter.

The NIH-Harvard experience

Pioneering work in this field—but with significant differences—has also been carried out in the United States. Considerable success has been achieved in monkeys, and a trial in a selected group of human transplant recipients is planned. Successful induction of tolerance in rodents was initially obtained by immunologist David Sachs and his colleagues at the National Institutes of Health (NIH) in Bethesda. Subsequent work by his group at Massachusetts General Hospital in Boston has led to collaborative studies in primates directed by Harvard transplant surgeon Ben Cosimi. In these studies, a monkey is treated with a combination of therapies. Important components include irradiation of the bone marrow, which is the site of blood cell production, and cytotoxic drugs to destroy the existing T lymphocytes. The thymus gland in the chest, which is the most important organ in the body involved in the "programming" of T lymphocytes to differentiate between self and non-self, is also irradiated. The purpose of this therapeutic package is to temporarily destroy the existing immune system, except for primitive cells that will recover and develop a new immune system. However, even this therapy is insufficient to ensure tolerance of an organ grafted at this time. Something more is required, and that something is a bone marrow transplant from the same donor as the organ.

During this period of immune paralysis, the recipient monkey is given an infusion of bone marrow cells from the prospective donor monkey. These bone marrow cells include many primitive cells that will mature into various cell types, some of which will form part of the new immune system of the host. Acceptance of this bone marrow transplant by the recipient results in the monkey now having a "chimeric" immune system—two systems working harmoniously together, its own (which has recovered) and that of the donor. The existence of these two immune systems in turn results in the development of tolerance to any organ or tissue subsequently grafted from that individual donor monkey. Kidney transplants in monkeys so treated have survived for years without any additional intervention. There have been no signs of the development of chronic rejection, and the monkeys retain a normal immune response to any invading microorganisms. Their immune systems appear to be fully intact except for the fact that they do not reject their grafts.

This remarkable achievement has been followed recently by an attempt to induce tolerance to xenografts, initially to kidneys from a closely related species (the baboon) and more recently from a distantly related species (the pig) (Figure 8.1). A small number of monkeys have received bone marrow and kidney transplants from baboons. Although chimerism was not uniformly achieved, in one or two cases the baboon kidney has survived for many months in the recipient monkey without further immunosuppressive drug therapy. The monkeys are active and in peak health, sustained only by baboon kidneys. If these studies can be extended to more distant species combinations, such as pig to primate, the development of tolerance to a kidney from another species would prove a major breakthrough in the field of xenotransplantation research.

The term "chimerism" has been adapted for use to describe the state achieved in these tolerance studies. The demonstration that donor bone mar-

figure 8.1. *One method being investigated of achieving immunological tolerance (or hyporesponsiveness) to a transplanted pig organ. First, the immune status of the recipient (in this case a baboon) is depleted by irradiation, drugs, and the immunoadsorption of anti-pig antibody from the blood. Pig bone marrow cells are then infused into the baboon's blood. If these pig cells engraft along with the recipient's own recovering cells, the recipient should then be able to receive any organ from the same donor pig without the need for any immunosuppressive drug therapy.*

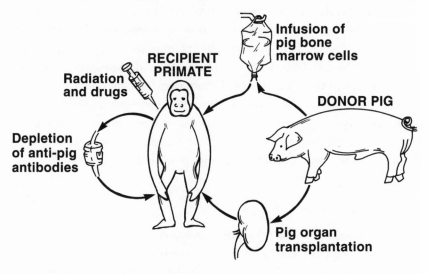

row cells survive alongside the recipient's own bone marrow cells has been termed "mixed chimerism," whether those donor bone marrow cells are from other human subjects or from another species. (Strictly speaking, all patients with organ transplants could be said to be chimeric, as they are made up of their own tissues plus the donor organ.)

Therapy involving a course of whole-body irradiation—necessary to deplete the immune system so that the donor marrow can take hold—seems quite drastic, and it places the patient at some risk. Following the course of irradiation, the numbers of white cells and platelets in the blood are reduced to extremely low levels for approximately one to two weeks. Since the white blood cells provide much of the body's protection against invading bacteria and other potentially infectious pathogens, the patient is at risk of developing serious infection during this period. The reduction of platelets puts the patient temporarily at risk from spontaneous bleeding. These risks can be minimized to some extent by antibiotic therapy and platelet transfusions.

Also, we now have much experience managing patients who have received even greater doses of whole-body radiation to received bone marrow transplants for the treatment of many malignant conditions, such as leukemia and metastasized cancer of the breast. The irradiation used in these cases is often combined with intensive chemotherapy and is intended to completely destroy the malignant cells, but in so doing it also kills healthy bone marrow cells, with no chance that those healthy cells will recover. A bone marrow transplant from a healthy human donor is therefore used to reconstitute a normal immune system.

A patient who has undergone a successful bone marrow transplant is therefore, like an organ recipient, technically considered chimeric (even though all of his/her bone marrow cells are from the same species, namely human). Once this chimeric state has been achieved, the patient could theoretically accept an organ, such as a kidney, from the same donor at any time in the future without the need for immunosuppressive drug therapy. Although this has been carried out successfully on rare occasions, it is unusual for a patient who requires a bone marrow transplant for malignant disease to also require a subsequent kidney or other solid organ transplant.

Can we learn to tolerate pigs?

The possibility of creating tolerance in baboons to pig organs is now under intense investigation. The major barrier is the presence of the anti-pig antibodies circulating in the bloodstream of the host. These cause rejection of the transplanted organ before tolerance can be induced. Although the suppression of the immune system by the radiation therapy is efficient in eliminating all of the T lymphocytes, it does not totally suppress the production of antibodies by the B lymphocytes and plasma cells. Plasma cells, in particular, are very resistant to irradiation. Anti-pig antibodies, therefore, remain active and lead to early graft rejection. If this problem can be overcome by the methods discussed in Chapter 6 (depletion and suppression of production of antibodies), then perhaps humans can be rendered tolerant to transplanted pig organs. This is the ultimate goal of many transplant surgeons and immunologists today.

The induction of tolerance depends on suppressing the T lymphocytes just long enough for the infused donor bone marrow to establish itself in the body. The reduction in antibody production depends on suppression of the B lymphocytes. To date, it has not proved possible to switch off anti-pig antibody production completely in baboons. However, Harvard immunologist Megan Sykes and her research group at Massachusetts General Hospital have demonstrated that this phenomenon is possible in rodents. This group has demonstrated that successful engraftment in the recipient of donor bone marrow cells that express a specific antigen leads to discontinuation of production of antibodies directed against that antigen. This has been achieved in Gal-knockout mice so that they no longer make anti-Gal antibodies. This means that the therapy administered to the recipient mice resulted in what is known as B-cell tolerance as well as T-cell tolerance.

B-cell tolerance, in which antibody production is completely suppressed and antibodies against the donor antigens are therefore absent, differs from the accommodation discussed in Chapter 6. In accommodation, the transplanted organ survives (for reasons we cannot explain) despite the presence of host antibodies directed against antigens on the organ cell surfaces.

The problems are not all immunological, however; they also include those of molecular incompatibility. Pig bone marrow cells, for example, do not proliferate well in the environment of human or baboon stroma (the background structural tissues that support the cells); the pig cells are stimulated to grow and proliferate by growth factors that are to some extent specific to pigs, and in the presence of baboon (or human) growth factors, they fare less well. To combat this problem, the Boston-based biotechnology company BioTransplant has developed pig-specific growth factors that stimulate pig bone marrow cell proliferation even in a human stromal environment.

There is, therefore, hope that we may be on the verge of achieving immunological tolerance, first to transplanted human organs and subsequently to pig organs.

Spontaneous Unresponsiveness o o o

Although tolerance has proved difficult to achieve by manipulation of the immune system at the time of the transplant, there is a small number of patients with human organ transplants who appear to have spontaneously developed a similar (but perhaps not identical) tolerant state. These few patients have generally been on immunosuppressant drugs for many years, but for one reason or another the drugs have been discontinued. In some cases they were slowly reduced by the attending physician over months or years and eventually discontinued entirely if the patient showed no signs of rejection. In other cases, they were withdrawn abruptly, perhaps because the patient was at risk of dying from overwhelming infection or cancer, and withdrawal was aimed at increasing the patient's resistance to the infection or malignant disease. There have even been cases when the drugs have been inadvertently (or purposely) discontinued by the patients themselves without the knowledge of their physicians. Whatever the reason for discontinuation, their bodies did not reject the transplanted organ. While again this state has been recorded in only a very small number of patients in comparison with the hundreds of thousands who have undergone organ transplantation during the past 40 years or so, there are occasional patients, particularly those with liver transplants, who have survived without taking any drugs for several years. It is almost certainly not true immunological tolerance, but rather a state of nonreactivity to the transplanted organ that has developed over many years. A second graft from the same donor, if this were possible, would probably be rejected, although we do not know this for certain. In a truly tolerant patient, a second graft from the same donor would be accepted. Furthermore, in the nonreactive patient (as opposed to the truly immunologically tolerant patient) it is likely that any rejection of the second graft would also cause simultaneous rejection of the first graft as well.

Molecular Chimerism: A New Concept o o o

There is one other, conceptually new approach that may give us the desired result of tolerance to pig organs. This approach is being explored by David Sachs and French molecular biologist Christian LeGuern at Massachusetts General Hospital in collaboration with scientists at Biotransplant. Rather than inducing mixed chimerism in the recipient by the introduction of donor cells, for example, pig bone marrow cells, the aim is to induce this state by the introduction of pig genes. This has been termed "molecular chimerism."

The Massachusetts General Hospital research group has the great advantage of working with a herd of miniature swine that have been carefully inbred over the past 20 years. As a result, strains have been developed with distinct tissue types. This is the only pig herd in the world where the range of tissue types between members of the herd is so restricted and so well defined. This inbreeding (and near identity of tissue type between many members of the herd) is proving invaluable in transplantation research. It is only by having access to such a herd that work on molecular chimerism can be undertaken.

The first step, which has been successfully achieved, is for the pig genes for the important tissue antigens to be cloned by molecular biological techniques. Bone marrow cells are then aspirated from the potential recipient baboon. In the laboratory, the pig gene (or genes) of interest is introduced into the bone marrow cells using retroviral technology. In this technology, the ability of a virus to penetrate the cell is utilized to carry the desired gene into the cell. The final step is for these gene-transduced cells to be reinfused back into the baboon. For the cells to engraft satisfactorily, the same course of therapy is given as for a pig bone marrow transplant. This includes whole body irradiation, as described above. Once the pig gene is expressed in the baboon, a kidney from a pig of the same tissue type is transplanted into the baboon. Preliminary testing indicates that although the presence of the gene does not inhibit the anti-Gal antibodies, it does inhibit the subsequent T-cell-induced rejection response. Once again, it is the antibodies that are proving the stumbling block.

But even this hurdle may be overcome by the introduction of yet another pig gene—the gene that leads to the production of the Gal sugar, namely, the gene for the enzyme GT. Encouraging preliminary studies have recently been carried out in Gal-knockout mice by Harvard scientist John Iacomini and his group. As Gal-knockout mice produce anti-Gal antibodies, they reject organ or cell transplants from normal (wild-type) mice, which express the Gal sugar on their cell surfaces. The introduction of the GT gene into Gal-knockout mice led to the presence of this enzyme and the production of the Gal sugar in the mouse's own cells. The presence of the sugar led the mouse to suppress production of anti-Gal antibody—evidently the mouse's body tried to avoid destroying its own cells even if they did express Gal. Wild-type mouse bone marrow cells subsequently intravenously infused into the Gal-knockout mouse were not rejected, as the mouse no longer had antibodies that could destroy these cells. B-cell tolerance had been successfully induced.

The pig GT gene has now been successfully expressed in baboon bone marrow cells. The presence of this gene in the baboon cells initiates production of Gal. After irradiation of the baboon, these Gal-producing bone marrow cells are infused back into the animal. The baboon's immune system is tricked into believing that the Gal sugar is "self" and, as in the Gal-knockout mice, it will not wish to destroy its own cells. These experiments are still too preliminary to lead to any definite conclusions, but it is hoped that the presence of the sugar on the baboon's own cells will result in deletion or suppression of the B lymphocytes that make Gal-reactive antibodies. If this happens, molecular chimerism may resolve the critical problem of antibody-mediated rejection of pig organs.

The Induction of Chimerism Before Birth:
Science Fiction or the Future of Transplantation? o o o

We offer one final thought on achieving tolerance to an organ graft, which is not likely for the present but may prove the ultimate goal of transplant surgeons at some future date. The association between bone marrow chimerism (i.e., an animal that has and tolerates cells both from itself and from a bone marrow donor) and tolerance of a transplanted skin or organ graft was actually reported as long ago as the late 1940s and early 1950s. American scientist Ray Owen was the first to describe chimerism of red blood cells in what are known as freemartin cattle. Freemartin cattle are fraternal (nonidentical) twins that share a common blood supply during life in the womb. Owen observed that exchange of blood between the twins' circulation before birth led to the development of stable, lifelong blood cell chimerism in both animals. In other words, each twin had some of its own and some of its twin's blood cells. Shortly thereafter, the British immunologist and Nobel laureate Sir Peter Medawar noted that skin grafts from one Freemartin twin to its sibling were permanently accepted and never rejected, whereas skin grafts from other cattle in the herd were rejected normally. Medawar hypothesized that the sharing of the blood cells (mixed blood cell chimerism) in some way permitted this donor-specific graft acceptance (or immunological tolerance).

The intravenous injection of white blood cells from another human or a pig into an unmodified adult human generally causes sensitization (or immunization) of the recipient by stimulating the production of antibodies against that donor. An organ subsequently grafted from the same donor might well be rejected hyperacutely by an antibody-mediated response. However, if these cells are injected into a fetus at the right time during pregnancy, they have the opposite effect: they cause tolerance, not sensitization. A subsequent organ graft from the same donor at any time, even well after birth, is then accepted permanently. This is because, if the cells are injected before the immune system is fully developed, the body cannot differentiate the cells of the donor from its own cells, and therefore treats them as "self." In contrast to achieving tolerance in an adult, in the fetus it is not necessary to give any course of irradiation or drugs to suppress and deplete the immune system, as it is still "naive."

In mice this state of tolerance can be achieved when blood cells are shared throughout fetal life and even up to about 72 hours after birth. Unfortunately, in humans the sharing of cells has to take place early in the pregnancy. The human fetus develops a competent immune system by about the end of the fourth month. Therefore, the introduction of any new cells has to be carried out before this occurs. After the fourth month, the newly introduced cells will be recognized as foreign. This knowledge might allow us to prepare humans to accept pig organs without the need for any form of therapy. However, this would necessitate the injection of pig cells into the human fetus during the early weeks of life in the womb which, with current techniques, might well be hazardous to the developing infant, and could lead to miscarriage. Since we cannot predict who might require a pig organ transplant, all human fetuses would have to be "tolerized" in this way for the procedure to be of benefit.

This form of mass "tolerization" may not be ethically acceptable today (and in any case is not yet technically possible). But, when the xenotransplantation of organs is established on a regular basis, the concept will almost certainly be fully explored. If the developing infant could be made tolerant without harmful effects, at some stage in the future all developing babies may be injected with pig cells to ensure that they could undergo pig organ transplantation in later life. Although this may currently be perceived to be science fiction, some research groups are already actively exploring this method of tolerance induction in experimental animals. But is it really very different from what we do today to immunize infants against diseases such as whooping cough and measles? Less than 75 years ago, a mother would have been amazed, and maybe even resistant, if it had been suggested that her newborn baby should be immunized against certain infections for which the child might (or might not) be at risk in the future. Today immunization against infections is readily accepted by the vast majority of the worldwide community. In the future, tolerance induction for subsequent pig transplants may become equally acceptable.

chapter 9

From Diabetes to Alzheimer's

Cells that will make a difference

Sweet Success: Cell Transplants for Diabetes ○ ○ ○

The child is too young to understand the concept of diabetes, or to realize that her parents are not trying to punish her. She had been sent home from school earlier in the day because the glucose levels in her blood were out of control. For the second time that afternoon, her mother, a nurse, is trying to get her to cooperate. As she pokes the needle into the child's arm—already badly bruised—to administer insulin, the child breaks into tears and asks: "Mommy, why do you hate me so much?"

This little girl is fortunate in that she has a mother who will ensure that her diabetes is controlled as well as possible. Nevertheless, in the coming decades she may develop one or more of the long-term degenerative complications of diabetes mellitus: an increased risk of going blind, of developing kidney failure, of having a heart attack or a stroke, or of needing to have a gangrenous limb amputated due to advanced vascular disease. Sadly, until now, the prospect of a cure for her disease has been slim and, despite hundreds of millions of dollars of research, there has essentially been no new therapy for diabetes since insulin was discovered by Nobel laureates Sir Frederick Banting and John Macleod and their junior colleague, Charles Best, over 75 years ago.

The transplantation of small clusters of pancreatic cells—called the islets of Langerhans after the scientist who first described them in 1869—may soon change all this. An increasing body of evidence regarding the transplantation of these insulin-producing cells in animals indicates that methods for successful xenografting of islets in diabetic patients are being developed and will be tested during the next several years.

Children and young adults have diabetes of the Type I, or insulin-dependent, form, in which there is a marked decrease in the number of insulin-producing cells in the pancreas compared with healthy individuals. In the past, and indeed even today, animal (usually pig or cow) or recombinant human sources of insulin, injected regularly, have provided the replacement therapy that is required on a day-to-day basis by these patients for survival. Unfortunately, injected insulin cannot precisely mimic the ability of the normal pancreas to continuously regulate blood sugar concentrations. The cells in the body need insulin in order to take up sugar from the blood to provide energy for them to function. The concentration of insulin in the blood is normally reciprocally linked to the blood sugar concentration by moment-to-moment fluctuations in insulin secretion by the pancreatic islets in response to food intake. These fluctuations in insulin secretion, which serve to control blood sugar concentrations, are dependent upon a complex series of biochemical pathways in the islet cell, and are extremely difficult or impossible to simulate by insulin injection. If too little insulin is injected, the sugar can accumulate to a high level, leading to a chemical imbalance that has profound effects on the body's metabolism. If too much insulin is administered, the blood sugar concentration rapidly drops to a dangerously low level, resulting in confusion, coma, and even death.

The results of the Diabetes Control and Complications Trial, carried out at several dozen centers in the United States and Canada from 1983 to 1993, indicated that failure to achieve physiological glucose control with injected insulin is responsible for the long-term complications of this disease, such as blindness. Since the transplantation of islets would restore proper physiological insulin production and maintain sugar values within normal limits at all times, there is hope that this form of therapy will not only eliminate the need for regular insulin injections, but prove effective in preventing or retarding the development of the various chronic diabetes-related ills.

The young Type I diabetic, of whom there are an estimated 600,000 to 1 million in the United States alone, forms only part of the overall picture of diabetes. Older people may develop a less aggressive form of the disease, known as Type II diabetes. There are an estimated 15 million such patients in the United States, 140 million worldwide, and the number is increasing by 2% per year. It has been estimated that at least one new person is diagnosed with diabetes every 60 seconds. The blood sugar of most of these patients can be controlled satisfactorily by attention to diet alone, but some 15 to 20%

(at least 2 million people in the United States) require insulin injections. The demand for transplantation of islet cells, if this could be achieved success- fully, would therefore probably dwarf the demand for any of the whole-organ grafts we have considered elsewhere in this volume.

Unfortunately, like other human organs, donor pancreases are in short supply. In the United States, only approximately 2,000 pancreases are recov- ered from cadavers each year; the rate of procurement is low partly because relatively few transplant centers have expertise in pancreas transplantation. Even with improved procurement of human organs, the supply of donor tis- sue would remain ridiculously inadequate if pancreatic islet transplantation were to be developed as an effective therapy. Furthermore, as the islet cells comprise only 1–2% of the volume of the pancreas, and some of these are lost during islet isolation and preparation, the islets from more than one pancreas (usually three to eight) may be required to treat just one diabetic patient.

For the immediate future, the logical alternative is to use nonhuman donor islets. Methods—largely a combination of mechanical disruption and enzymatic digestion—have been developed to isolate islets from pig and cow pancreatic glands. These provide an attractive option because the amino acid sequences of their insulins are similar to those of human insulin. Indeed, insulins from these animals are fully active in humans and have been used to treat diabetics for over 75 years. There would be no restriction on the supply of pancreases from these species, which are obviously readily avail- able in very large numbers.

Islet transplants

In the late 19th century, nearly three decades before the discovery of in- sulin, ambitious and innovative physicians in the British city of Bristol at- tempted to treat a diabetic child by injecting fragments from the pancreas of a sheep. The procedure did not prove successful. There were no further reports of clinical islet xenotransplantation until the mid-1980s, when fetal pancreatic tissue from pigs and cows was transplanted into patients in Moscow and Kiev and, more recently, in Stockholm and Auckland. Islets taken from animal fetuses have some advantages over more mature cells in that they grow more rapidly in culture and are more amenable to prepa- ration and storage.

Detailed scientific information is available from the Swedish study, headed by Carl Groth of the Karolinska Institute. Fetal pig islets were trans- planted into 10 diabetic patients, being injected either into a vein that carried them into the liver or directly under the capsule surrounding the kidney, both sites where they are known to be able to survive and grow. These patients had either received (human) kidney transplants previously or had a kidney transplanted at the time the islet cells were injected. All were therefore on a regimen of immunosuppressive drugs. Samples of islet tissue (biopsies) taken three weeks after transplantation revealed viable insulin-positive cells in two of the patients. Although pig C-peptide (a measure of insulin synthesis) could be detected in the serum and urine of the patients for several months, the transplanted islet cells had little or no impact on the amount of injected insulin needed to control their diabetes. The trial could therefore not be considered a success.

A similar trial at Auckland Children's Hospital in New Zealand involved six young diabetic patients. "Naked" or unprotected pig islets were transplanted into four, and encapsulated islets into two. Although one patient's insulin requirement fell by 30%, overall the trial was no more successful than that in Sweden.

Overcoming islet rejection

The above studies draw attention to the major problem of rejection of islets, both those derived from humans as well as those derived from animals. Although transplanting islet cells requires only a simple injection, which is clearly preferable to the surgical procedure required to transplant the whole pancreas, human islet cells are exquisitely sensitive to rejection and may also be damaged by autoimmune activity specifically directed against them. Indeed, some cases of the original diabetes itself result from autoimmune injury, where the body's immune system injures its own cells. As a result, the success of even human islet transplantation has been sporadic, and the need for immunosuppressive drug therapy, to prevent both rejection and autoimmune injury, exposes these patients (as with other organ transplant recipients) to a wide variety of complications. In addition, some of the immunosuppressive drugs used, including steroids and cyclosporine, themselves have a direct deleterious effect on islet cell function and on glucose control. However, researchers are confident that with the introduction of new techniques and new immunosuppressive agents, successful human islet transplantation will eventually prove consistently successful. But the problem of inadequate supply of human pancreases will remain.

The hyperacute rejection that destroys pig organs may be avoided when pig islets are transplanted. Islet cell preparations, as well as many of the other cell preparations discussed in this chapter, are frequently devoid of blood vessels. New blood vessels have to grow into them from the host. They may therefore be relatively low in expression of the important Gal sugar. Although this factor may give them some resistance to hyperacute rejection, they are still rejected within days by a poorly understood rejection response.

However, a practical means for evading the rejection of animal cells without immunosuppression is already undergoing clinical trial. This strategy—known as immunoisolation—not only is being used to protect transplanted islet cells from rejection, but can also be employed to protect other types of cells or small packages of tissues.

Solitary confinement

Several different types of immunoisolation systems have been developed and studied during the past several years. In all of these systems, the basic premise is that transplanted cells are physically separated from the hostile immunological environment of the host by encapsulation in a synthetic, selectively-permeable membrane. Small molecules, such as nutrients, oxygen, and certain therapeutic agents, can cross the membrane, while large molecules, such as antibodies and white blood cells (which are the two main culprits in rejection), are blocked from doing so (Figures 9.1 and 9.2). Although this strategy does not address the needs of patients who require whole organs, it nevertheless has enormous potential value in treating patients who suffer tissue loss or cellular dysfunction and therefore require transplants only of cells. In addition, cells and tissues offer several advantages over whole organs in other respects. They can be biologically manipulated comparatively easily and can be maintained outside of the body to allow preparation or storage for longer periods than are possible when working with intact organs.

Indeed, the ability to manipulate cells in culture in the laboratory—by introducing new genes or knocking out unwanted genes—and to reproduce the modified cells in large numbers by cloning will open up enormous potential in the treatment of many disease processes. Notwithstanding an ability to clone whole animals, such as the famous sheep Dolly, the rapid cloning of manipulated cells may prove the major and lasting contribution of this new technology.

The approach of immunoisolation has broad application in the treatment not only of diabetes but of a wide range of other disorders, including the use of liver cells for the treatment of liver failure, chromaffin cells for chronic pain, and cells that produce blood-clotting factors for hemophilia or nerve growth factors for neurodegenerative disorders such as Parkinson's and Alzheimer's diseases. Moreover, by using recombinant DNA and cell enfigure **9.1.** *Drawing of how transplanted encapsulated porcine islet cells can release insulin into the circulation and yet be protected from the destructive effects of the patient's immune response.*

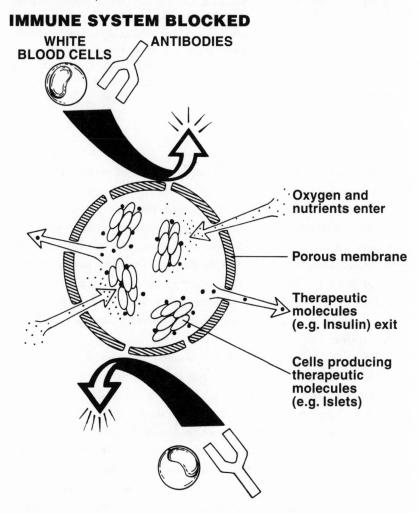

IMMUNE SYSTEM BLOCKED

WHITE BLOOD CELLS

ANTIBODIES

Oxygen and nutrients enter

Porous membrane

Therapeutic molecules (e.g. Insulin) exit

Cells producing therapeutic molecules (e.g. Islets)

gineering technologies, it may also prove possible to treat patients suffering from immunodeficiency states and even cancer.

Although human clinical trials using encapsulated animal cells for the treatment of chronic pain, liver failure, and amyotrophic lateral sclerosis (Lou Gehrig's disease) have already been initiated, to date most research involving immunoisolation has been carried out with pancreatic islet cells. Perfused devices (large sheathed implants connected to a supply of blood), hollow plastic fibers or chambers unconnected to the bloodstream, and small in-

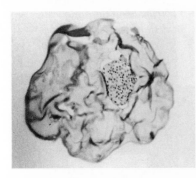

figure 9.2. *Encapsulated insulin-producing pancreatic islet cells from the pig may eventually serve to produce insulin in patients afflicted with diabetes. The biodegradable polymer membrane surrounding the islets allows secreted insulin to pass through it, but protects the islets from attack by components of the patient's immune system. (See Figure 9.1, p. 125.)*

jectable alginate gel capsules (or microspheres) are all in various stages of development and trial.

Perfused devices containing isolated cow or pig islet cells have been used successfully in diabetic dogs, which have exhibited substantially reduced insulin requirement for up to nine months. Despite this promise, there are several disadvantages to this approach. Most important, the patient requires major surgery for implantation of the device, which involves direct connection of the device to the patient's blood vessels. And because it is continuously being perfused by blood, the device is always at risk from being occluded by clots.

Engineering and implanting hollow plastic fibers or chambers to isolate cells from the recipient's immune system has also proved successful in rodents and dogs. Using these systems, pig, cow, and dog islets have restored blood sugar levels in diabetic rats for more than a year without the use of immunosuppressive drugs. While these chambers appear to have solved the problem of rejection of xenogeneic cells in rodents, studies in large animals phylogenetically closer to humans will be required before clinical trials in humans can be initiated. Preliminary experiments have, in fact, already been performed in diabetic dogs, but in these studies canine islet allografts (rather than xenografts) were tested. Whereas prior to implantation of the device the dog's daily insulin requirements ranged from 30 to 40 units per day, which is in the range of what most human patients require, after implantation insulin injections were no longer necessary. However, although the surgery to implant such chambers is minor compared with the implantation of a perfused device, it remains unclear how well patients would tolerate the long-term presence of the implanted plastic materials or the need for replacement with "fresh" devices fairly frequently, which is likely to be a requirement of long-term islet replacement therapy.

In an effort to overcome the difficulties and potential complications in-

herent in the implantation of plastic fibers or perfused devices, a new technology has recently been introduced in which the islets are encased in small
biodegradable capsules that can simply be injected under the skin or into the
abdominal cavity with a syringe (see Figure 9.2). One gram of islets from pigs,
containing at least one million islets, should be sufficient to supply the needs
of the average diabetic patient.

Encapsulated islets from cows have remained alive and functional in
dogs for six weeks, the point at which the test was concluded. These studies,
and others in diabetic mice, rats, and rabbits, suggest that encapsulated pig
islets would most likely survive in human patients for from several months
to more than a year. Eventually, the tiny packages would degrade, so no
surgery will be required to remove the old capsules when the supply of islet
cells needs to be replenished. New capsules and cells will simply be injected.
Clinical trials of this technique are planned to begin soon, and could lead
the way to a better life for the world's many diabetic patients.

Reversing a Jaundiced View of the World: Cell Transplants for Liver Failure ○ ○ ○

The 51-year-old grandmother had recently moved to the Gulf coast of Mississippi from Illinois. It was a special day, and she was preparing breaded
and deep-fried wild mushrooms as a novelty dish for her family's Sunday
brunch. Mushroom hunting was a popular pastime with her, and she had
accumulated over three decades of expertise in selecting and preparing wild
mushroom dishes. However, it was her husband who had gathered the mushrooms the day before—and he had collected only the caps, leaving the stems
in the ground. She therefore had no idea that the mushrooms were of the
Amanita genus (which have a skirtlike ring at the top of the stalk and a pouch
at the base). From what she could see, they looked just like an edible mushroom that grew in the woodlands of her native state. Unfortunately, *Amanita*
mushrooms contain one of the most deadly liver toxins known.

About 12 hours after she served brunch, four of the five family members
presented to the emergency room of the local hospital with nausea, cholera-
like diarrhea and abdominal cramps. According to the medical report in *The
American Journal of Gastroenterology*, in 1995, liver enzyme abnormalities
were recognized. The three adults were successfully treated with intravenous
fluids, electrolyte repletion, and activated charcoal. Unfortunately, her three-
year-old granddaughter continued to deteriorate. By the fourth day, the child
was transferred to a transplant center, where she was listed for an emergency
liver transplant. The next day she went into a deep coma and required ven-

tilator support. A few days later she died from irreversible liver failure complicated by pneumonia and infection.

It is accepted that the heart and brain are essential to our survival, but the liver is equally essential, although death occurs more slowly if the liver stops functioning than if the heart does. The liver is responsible for a myriad of complex biochemical activities, including the metabolism of dietary protein, fats, and carbohydrates, the production of numerous hormones and enzymes, and the removal of toxins from the blood, all processes which are essential for the maintenance of life. Failure of the organ can therefore clearly be life-threatening.

Current therapy

As we have discussed elsewhere in this volume, there is currently no adequate therapy for severe liver failure. Rapid or fulminant liver failure, which most commonly results from viral infection (hepatitis) or from consumed chemical toxins (which can sometimes include certain prescription drugs, such as acetaminophen), has a high mortality rate of between 70 and 95%. It accounts for about 2,000 deaths in the United States and almost 300 in the United Kingdom each year. Death is usually from a combination of swelling of the brain and failure of other vital organs, which all depend in one way or another on the adequate function of the liver. In extreme cases, death may occur within hours.

Although numerous attempts have been made to treat liver failure using artificial support systems, such as charcoal hemoperfusion (perfusion of blood over charcoal, which adsorbs out certain toxins), hemodialysis, hemofiltration, and plasma exchange, none of these strategies has succeeded in improving patient survival significantly. The average hospital stay in the United States for a patient with fulminant hepatic failure is 14 days and costs $74,000 (exclusive of physicians' fees). The average cost would be much higher were it not for the sad fact that 75% of the patients die in the hospital soon after admission.

At present, liver transplantation is the only therapeutic option in patients with irreversible liver disease. However, the surgical procedure is formidable, the post-transplant period can be complicated, and there remains the major problem of the limited availability of human donor livers. As an alternative to whole-liver transplantation, investigators are now studying the transplantation of "naked" pig liver cells (hepatocytes) or, more commonly, of immunoisolated hepatocytes, not only for the treatment of irreversible liver failure but also for several other deficiency states or disease processes. These include hereditary enzyme abnormalities in which the liver is unable to produce essential or important enzymes.

In addition, transplanted pig hepatocytes might act as a temporary "bridge" to whole-liver transplantation in patients who develop sudden liver failure. The cell infusion requires minimal surgical intervention and would therefore be suitable for use in very sick patients. Furthermore, the therapy does not entail removal of the patient's own liver, and would therefore allow recovery or regeneration of the liver whenever this may be a possibility.

The potential physiological and biochemical limitations of pig liver transplantation apply equally to the transplantation of pig liver cells. First, the pig hepatocytes will be producing pig complement, not human complement, which may have a detrimental immunological effect on some of the human recipient's own cells and tissues. This is an area about which virtually nothing is known to date. Will we be faced by some new form of graft-versus-host disease, which has proved a major problem after bone marrow transplantation? (When bone marrow cells are transplanted into a recipient depleted of all immune cells, the donor T cells can actually begin to reject some of the host tissues. This is particularly problematic in the skin and bowel, and may indeed prove fatal.) The production of pig complement may lead to a complement-induced (rather than a T-cell-induced) form of graft-versus-host disease, which we have never seen previously.

Second, the pig enzymes, hormones, proteins, and other bioactive substances produced by the hepatocytes may be structurally and functionally different enough from their human counterparts to prevent their being useful. Indeed, they may be sufficiently different to stimulate the recipient's immune system to make antibodies against them and thus neutralize their effects. Antibodies may also develop against pig complement, further complicating the picture.

Nevertheless, even with these reservations, the infusion of pig hepatocytes may be useful in several conditions for which current therapeutic options are lamentably inadequate. In particular, the detoxifying functions of the pig liver may be sufficient to support a dying human patient until his/her liver failure spontaneously recovers or is cured by a liver transplant.

Patients with long-standing (chronic) liver failure, however, will require protracted functional support by the transplanted cells, which makes them much less suitable for this form of therapy. Methods of isolating, transplanting, and maintaining very large numbers of cells would be required. Hepatocytes are difficult to culture in the laboratory, but have been shown to function better when they are immobilized in physiological matrices, such as collagen, microcarriers, or alginate. Therefore, researchers are now trying to develop liver support systems (both implantable and external) that combine isolated hepatocytes with artificial materials and mechanical components. For example, several groups have attempted to develop microencapsulation of liver cells and have demonstrated the viability and regeneration of such encapsulated cells after transplantation in rodent models.

Bioartificial livers

Although patients with failing kidneys can be supported for many years by renal dialysis, and patients with advanced heart failure can be supported, at least for several months, by left ventricular assist devices and other forms of artificial heart, there is no truly successful means of supporting a patient with advanced liver failure. However, hepatic equivalents of kidney dialysis, known as extracorporeal liver assist devices (ELADs) or bioartificial livers, are being developed. It has been estimated that as many as 80,000 patients worldwide might benefit from such devices each year. Although numerous systems of cell-based ELADs have been studied in the laboratory, only a few designs have successfully reached evaluation in patients so far.

The ideal ELAD needs to provide at least 30% of the function of a healthy liver. This translates into an ELAD containing about 5 billion hepatocytes. The cells that constitute the device can be freshly isolated from a healthy liver (human or animal) or, alternatively, obtained from cells in continuous culture, that is, cloned or immortalized liver cells, possibly from a liver tumor. Freshly isolated cells have some disadvantages; most notably, they do not divide and proliferate well, which makes it difficult to obtain them in the numbers required for repeated treatments.

A successful ELAD needs sufficient metabolic capacity, should ideally provide continuous liver support, must be available at short notice, and should be easy to operate. The safety of the device is also important, but as the patients being treated have a risk of dying from fulminant liver failure approaching 90%, it is clear that some risk may be ethically acceptable.

Trials in patients have been sporadic. In 1987, researchers in Berkeley, California, used a device containing a suspension of rabbit hepatocytes to treat a 45-year-old man, who recovered sufficiently to be discharged from the hospital. There have, however, been no further reports on the development of this system. In 1989, doctors in Latvia treated 59 patients with liver failure using a device containing a suspension of pig hepatocytes and activated charcoal. Sixty-three percent of the patients survived, compared with only 41% in a control group of 67 patients who received standard medical therapy.

In the early 1990s, using a microporous hollow-fiber bioreactor seeded with pig hepatocytes, Achilles Demetriou and his colleagues at the Cedars-Sinai Medical Center in Los Angeles treated nine patients with fulminant liver failure. Eight either recovered completely or were successfully bridged to liver transplantation. The Cedars-Sinai team then joined efforts with the giant chemical and medical company W. R. Grace & Co. to further develop this hollow-fiber ELAD. (W. R. Grace & Co. created a new business unit called Circe Biomedical, which is now an independent private company.) Isolated pig hepatocytes were attached to collagen-coated microcarriers and inoculated into the chamber outside of the hollow fibers through which the patient's plasma would circulate (Figures 9.3 and 9.4). Several thousand of the hollow fiber tubes are present within a plastic cartridge.

Two groups of patients were treated with the ELAD for seven-hour periods on one or more occasions. The first group consisted of 11 patients who were awaiting a liver transplant, 10 of whom were in deep coma from fulminant liver failure. Treatment resulted in a significant improvement in their neurological status, and all were successfully bridged to liver transplantation and were eventually discharged from the hospital with full neurological recovery. The second group consisted of eight patients with long-standing liver disease who were not candidates for transplantation, but who were suffering

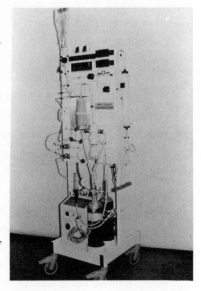

figure 9.3. *The Circe HepatAssist 2000 extracorporeal liver assist device (artificial liver). (Courtesy of Claudy Mullon, Ph.D., Circe Biomedical Inc., Lexington, MA.)*

figure 9.4. *The Circe HepatAssist 2000 liver assist device (artificial liver) consists of a bioartificial liver cartridge (on the left) coupled to a plasmapheresis system. The plasma is separated from the cellular components of the patient's blood and is passed through the cartridge. The liver cells "detoxify" the plasma of noxious substances that the patient's own liver is failing to remove.*

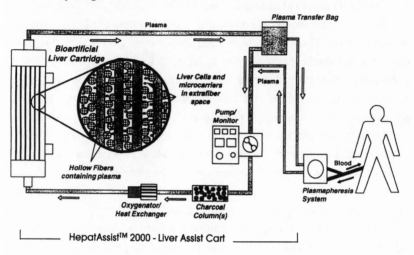

a rapid deterioration in their liver failure. Therapy was less successful; although all experienced at least transient beneficial effects from the ELAD, six died due to the failure of their livers to regenerate or recover. In total, over 50 patients have now been treated using the Circe Biomedical HepatAssist device at centers in Los Angeles and Paris. Fifteen percent of the patients recovered native liver function, and 70% went on to human liver transplantation. Overall survival has been almost 80%.

Even if these ELADs could only be used on one occasion, and then the cells needed to be changed, the ready availability of pig livers and therefore of pig hepatocytes, and probable low cost, would still make this a feasible method of treating patients with liver failure.

In the future, ELADs may be made up of cells from transgenically modified pigs or of cells that have been genetically manipulated and then cloned. This might further protect the cells from injury by the immune system. (In the United States, the FDA has approved one such clinical trial where, although an ELAD will not be used, the patient's blood will be perfused extracorporeally through livers from pigs transgenic for human complement regulatory proteins.) With time, it is possible that ELAD therapy may become the definitive treatment for fulminant hepatic failure, and may be able to support others waiting for a liver transplant.

The Brain: The Final Frontier? o o o

The "shaking palsy": Parkinson's disease

She had her whole life ahead of her. She was well and carefree until her 25th birthday, when she noted a tendency to drag her feet. After being diagnosed with early-onset Parkinson's disease, the young woman was treated with the drug levodopa, with good response for several years. She then started to develop the symptoms that are familiar to every doctor: stooped posture, blank, unemotional, or "masked" face, stiffness and slowness of movement, small voice, shuffling steps. The disease continued to progress, and she became so severely disabled that she could not walk even when assisted. She died at the age of 43 from a breathing impairment associated with her disease.

Unless a new treatment is found, approximately 500,000 people in the United States alone will be faced to a greater or lesser degree by the problems associated with the disease. Parkinson's disease, named after the early-19th-century British physician James Parkinson, who described it, is caused by the degeneration of a small group of cells in the brain that produce the hormone dopamine. Absence of dopamine, or low levels of it, result in weakness, tremors, and disordered movements that, in the late stages, alternate with a paralyzing immobility. Replacement therapy with drugs such as levodopa is available, but in many patients a point is eventually reached where pharmacotherapy can no longer compensate for the loss of brain cell activity.

Recent surgical treatment has focused on attempts to repair the defective region of the brain with cell grafts. The purpose is to transplant healthy brain cells into the diseased brain in the hope that the connections (synapses) between these healthy cells and the patient's own brain cells (neurons) will develop. Thus dopamine will be delivered in a regulated fashion via these connections. Alternatively, the dopamine may reach the synapses by simple diffusion. Other transplant strategies being tested include the implantation of cells producing trophic factors (growth or stimulatory factors) that may prevent the degeneration of the patient's own dopamine-producing nerve cells. More remarkably, the implantation of the specialized Sertoli cells from the testis has been demonstrated in animal models of Parkinson's disease to produce recovery of brain function, possibly by promoting growth of key structures in the recipient's brain or even by having a local immunosuppressive effect.

Human fetal cells: a present-day controversy

In both rodent and nonhuman primate models of Parkinson's disease, the transplantation of fetal dopamine-producing neurons has been shown to reinstate near-normal dopamine innervation and reduce abnormalities of muscular function in the limbs. Fetal brain cells, as with fetal pancreatic islet cells, have certain advantages over adult brain cells. In particular, fetal neuronal tissue is much more likely to grow and develop branching fibers, and is less likely to stimulate the recipient's immune response. Studies in rodents have demonstrated that fetal brain cell grafts become integrated into the brain of the recipient animal on a long-term basis, and can thus become a permanent functional part of the host animal. The transplanted cells send branches, or axons, into the host brain; these synthesize and release dopamine, and they form new synapses with the host's own neurons. The behavioral and functional manifestations seen in the disease can thus be reversed or, at least, alleviated.

Clinical trials using human fetal tissue have been carried out in over 200 patients with Parkinson's disease worldwide. Evidence of tissue survival and function for periods of more than a year has been accumulated. Carefully performed quantitative tests carried out by expert neurologists have documented a significant decrease in limb rigidity and increased speed of movement of the arms, hands, and feet. A greatly improved response to drug treatment has also been observed.

Neurosurgeons Thomas Freeman and Paul Sanberg and their associates at the University of South Florida transplanted human fetal cells into several patients, who subsequently received immunosuppressive drugs for six months. One of the patients died from an unrelated cause 18 months after the cell transplant, during which period he had shown a considerable degree of clinical improvement. Examination of the brain revealed excellent survival of the grafted cells, with more than 200,000 dopamine-producing neurons being identified. Furthermore, the cells were well integrated into the host's brain structure.

These and other exploratory studies suggest that the transplantation of dopamine-producing cells may become a safe and effective therapy for patients with Parkinson's disease. However, all of the donor tissues used in the above studies were obtained from aborted human fetuses, which is in itself a controversial, even explosive issue. But even if fetal cell research were not mired in political and ethical controversy, the fact that the cells from five or more intact fetuses are required to treat just one Parkinson's patient would make it impossible to obtain enough human tissue in this way to meet the demands of all potential patients.

However, the exciting new area of stem cell research could change all this. As discussed earlier, stem cells—usually derived from embryos and fetuses—have the potential to develop into any of the myriad cell types found in the body. Researchers at both Johns Hopkins University and the University of Wisconsin in Madison have recently isolated human embryonic stem cells. These scientists not only persuaded the stem cells to divide indefinitely, but succeeded in coaxing them to differentiate into a wide variety of cell types, including gut, cartilage, bone, muscle, and neuronal cells. Stem cells may eventually provide scientists with an ability to grow replacement human organs and tissues at will. This will include the brain cells needed to treat Parkinson's disease.

The pig to the rescue

However, at present, the obvious solution to the problem is to use donor cells from pigs, not humans. Toward that end, the function of nonhuman donor brain cells has been successfully explored in various animal models of Parkinson's disease. Within the confines of the brain, the transplanted pig cells are relatively protected from the immune response of the human recipient, as the blood-brain barrier reduces the transplanted cells' susceptibility to attack by either host antibodies or T lymphocytes. Fetal pig implants can reduce the deficit associated with an almost complete loss of dopamine-producing neurons. Furthermore, fibers from the transplanted cells can survive and grow to join up with the patient's own nerve fibers, indicating that repair of the brain microcircuitry is possible using implanted animal cells.

The results of these preclinical animal studies prompted surgeons at the Lahey Clinic in Boston—collaborating with scientists at Diacrin, a local biotechnology company—to transplant nerve cells from pig fetuses into the brains of patients with advanced Parkinson's disease, the first patient being treated in 1995. To prevent rejection, the patients were given either standard immunosuppressive drugs or the donor cells themselves were pretreated with fragments of antibody that masked and therefore protected them. Early indications are that patients surgically treated in this way can benefit, as measured by various tests of voluntary movement. Some experienced reduction of—or even nearly complete relief from—muscular rigidity, and this improvement has been sustained for almost three years. One patient reportedly abandoned the wheelchair he had been forced to use for several years, and he took up golf. Postmortem analysis of tissue obtained from a patient who died from an unrelated cause seven months after transplantation has further documented long-term viability of the xenografted tissues (Figure 9.5). The

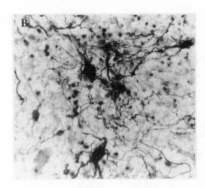

figure 9.5. *Clinical trials in which pig fetal nerve cells have been injected into the brains of patients with Parkinson's disease have indicated some success. In one patient, seven months later, pig cells (seen here in black) were documented to have survived and made connections with the patient's own brain cells. (Courtesy of Diacrin, Inc., Charlestown, Massachusetts. Reproduced with permission from* Nature Medicine 3, 350, 1997.)

neurosurgical team treating these patients is therefore optimistic that the pig can be used as a useful source of brain cells for transplantation.

The horizons expand: treating other neurological disorders with transplanted cells

More than 7 million patients in the United States suffer from other serious (non-Parkinson's) neurodegenerative disorders, such as Huntington's disease, amyotrophic lateral sclerosis (Lou Gehrig's disease), and Alzheimer's disease. A number of new compounds, called neurotrophic factors, have demonstrated in animal tests that they might be able to stem the degenerative effects caused by brain cell damage or disease. By implanting cells that secrete these trophic factors, scientists believe they can promote the survival and repair of cells whose degeneration leads not only to the above diseases but also to a number of other central and peripheral nervous system ailments.

Huntington's disease

He and his wife have agreed to be part of a medical workshop aimed at generating research on Huntington's disease. The man is gaunt and pale, with short, graying hair over a long face. His wife has the delicate frame of a songbird and is prim and neat in glasses and a green and white floral-print dress. They might be posing for a picture—a modern version of *American Gothic*—except that the man's body is constantly moving. He and his wife are politely being questioned by a roomful of doctors and biologists.

Thirteen years ago the man was diagnosed as having Huntington's disease, a rare neurological disorder (also known at Huntington's chorea) described in 1872 by the American physician George Huntington. The disease results from the degeneration of a specific set of brain neurons. As the nerve cells die, the disorder causes loss of thinking capacity (dementia) and rapid, uncontrollable movements of the joints and limbs. These irregular, jerking movements have a peculiar dancing quality to them. In fact, that is what the man is doing now. As the December 1993 issue of *Discover* magazine put it, "His hands dart and float in the air as if manipulated by an inebriated puppeteer. His head has a looseness that recalls those toy puppies whose heads once bobbed in the rear windows of American sedans. He watches his own limbs as if from a distance, occasionally reasserting control long enough to force a hand to grasp at the fabric of his pant leg or scratch the nape of his neck."

When the man first sought medical help, his symptoms consisted of irritability, lack of sleep, and "the jitters," but soon he began to lose his memory and became unable to work. The disease usually inexorably ravages both mind and body and leads to death about 15 years after the symptoms first appear. Patients not infrequently die choking on food they can no longer swallow. Because of its distressing and incapacitating nature, the suicide rate among Huntington's sufferers is seven times the United States national average.

Although there are only about 30,000 patients suffering from Huntington's disease in the United States, the disease has attracted much attention because, tragically, there is a 50% chance of a child of an affected parent being afflicted. There is currently no cure, nor even an effective treatment for preventing or slowing the relentless loss of neurons in the brain.

Transplantation of fetal tissue (from the area of the brain called the striatum) has been shown to produce behavioral improvements in animal models of Huntington's disease, and there are currently several ongoing trials in patients based on this approach, including one using pig fetal tissue. However, there are a number of obstacles to clinical application of this strategy. Unlike Parkinson's disease, where the transplanted cells need only deliver dopamine locally to produce a therapeutic benefit, the cell types that degenerate in Huntington's disease form important connections with other neurons in several different places in the brain. Unfortunately, the conditions for the reformation of these connections do not exist in adult patients, although transplanted fetal cells can form such synapses with the target cells. Therefore, rather than trying to replace the cells that have already been lost, some scientists are now studying the use of cells that produce trophic factors that might prevent further injury, or at least slow down the rate of destruction.

In rats, the neurotoxic effects of the drug quinolinic acid, which reproduces the pathology seen in Huntington's disease, have been shown to be attenuated by the transplantation of encapsulated fibroblasts that secrete nerve growth factor. Researchers at CytoTherapeutics in Rhode Island gave monkeys brain implants of encapsulated hamster kidney cells that had been genetically modified to produce another human neurotrophic factor, ciliary neurotrophic factor. A week later, the monkeys were given an injection of quinolinic acid. The implanted cells were found to exert a protective effect on nerve cells that were predicted to die following administration of the drug. These studies support the idea that trophic-factor-producing cells may help to prevent the degeneration of the various cell populations and circuits that form the basis of Huntington's disease.

Surgeons in both Boston and Florida have attempted treatment of a small number of patients using human and porcine fetal brain cells, but as yet it is too soon to assess their effect on the disease process.

Of baseball and black holes: the disease that killed Lou Gehrig

She is a middle-aged woman with amyotrophic lateral sclerosis—commonly referred to in the United States as Lou Gehrig's disease (after the famous American baseball player who was diagnosed with the disease during his playing days and succumbed to it two years later, in 1941). Lou Gehrig's disease is a frightening ailment characterized by the progressive degeneration of the motor neurons (nerve cells that control muscle movement), leaving its victims totally paralyzed. (Readers of the best-selling book *A Brief History of Time* may know that its author, Stephen Hawking, also has this disease. The quite remarkable Hawking, a theoretical physicist at the University of Cambridge in the United Kingdom and a world authority on the astronomical bodies known as black holes, is confined to a wheelchair and requires around-the-clock nursing care.)

At age 55, this woman, like Stephen Hawking, has lost the use of both arms and legs, cannot speak or eat solid foods, and cannot breathe normally. Her inability to carry out even the simplest task is evident from a letter she wrote to newspaper columnist Ann Landers (*Boston Globe*, August 7, 1997). She describes just how dependent she is on the generosity and support of friends: "Mary stepped in when my first two caregivers quit on short notice. She came to my apartment every night at 2 A.M. to turn me over. She also assisted with my personal correspondence and business. Lil assisted in my care and kept me company on many occasions. Mary Lee brought gifts to brighten my sickroom and read me books when I could no longer turn the pages. Bonnie brought special treats, shared her video collection and brought arrangements of lilacs, irises, and violets from her garden. Maria cooked my favorite meals and helped me continue entertaining guests in my apartment.

Kristin helped with correspondence and bookkeeping. Bruce picked up and returned my videotapes. Ray handled repairs and modifications to my apartment. These are just a few of the people who have made a difference in my life."

The course of the disease is relentlessly progressive, leading ultimately to death from respiratory failure due to loss of the nerves that control the diaphragm and muscles of the chest wall that enable us to breathe. The disease affects about 30,000 people in the United States, and more than half die within three years.

Ciliary neurotrophic factor has been shown to prevent such motor neuron loss in animal models of chronic nerve cell degeneration. Patrick Aebischer and his colleagues at the University of Lausanne in Switzerland have therefore initiated trials in patients using hamster cells in which the gene for human ciliary neurotrophic factor has been incorporated. By implanting chambers containing these cells in the lower spine, where the motor neurons degenerate, these investigators hope that they will have a beneficial effect on the course of the disease. No results are yet available.

The scourge of the aged—Alzheimer's disease

Former U.S. president Ronald Reagan is perhaps the most prominent of the estimated 4 million Americans who are afflicted with Alzheimer's disease, described in 1906 by a German psychiatrist and named after him. Alzheimer's is a degenerative disorder that affects the parts of the brain that control memory, language, and motor skills. An initial loss of memory proceeds to a progressive deterioration of many other mental functions. It is the commonest cause of dementia in the elderly, with all that this implies both economically and in terms of distress for patients with families. In the United States alone, it costs the health care system an estimated $80 billion to $100 billion a year!

Most of us know someone who has Alzheimer's disease. For example, in the July 1996 issue of *Ladies' Home Journal*, Lori Baker describes life with her mother, who over the last ten years has gradually lost her ability to function. She tells of how the disease has robbed them of the close relationship they once shared, how she has to feed, dress, and clean the woman who once did the same for her, how she has to answer the same questions again and again and again. Lori also describes the potential emergencies of which she and others like her live in fear. For instance, one woman's mother set her arm on fire while cooking, but had no idea how to put it out. Charles Pierce tells us in the February 1996 issue of *GQ* about his father, who forgot how to swallow, "so he breathed in his food" until it eventually killed him, and about his uncle (one of four brothers who developed Alzheimer's disease), a superbly educated priest, who one day simply forgot how to stand up.

Alzheimer's is clearly a devastating disease. Although it is incurable at present, recent experiments in animals offer hope. In rodents with memory impairment, the continuous infusion of nerve growth factor into the brain can prevent degeneration of neurons and is associated with improved cognitive function. Moreover, following treatment, the size of the key neurons increases, becoming closer to normal size for these animals. By implanting cells that secrete nerve growth factor or other neurotrophic factors, it may prove possible to prevent at least some of the neuronal deterioration that occurs in patients with Alzheimer's disease.

Epilepsy

Emma was born in a British mining village in 1953. Although her seizures started when she was only five years old, it wasn't until she left secondary school that her troubles really began. Unable to find a job, there was not much for her to do in the small village. At first she helped her mother in the house, but soon the seizures became more frequent. Her doctor increased her anticonvulsants, but the sedative effects of the drugs slowed her down and impaired her thinking. She made numerous visits to specialists and required hospital admissions. "On readmission," wrote one of her doctors (*Nursing Times*, September 19, 1974), "Emma had deteriorated pathetically. She was barely able to walk and her speech was very difficult to control. She was euphoric, sitting, smiling, giggling, making almost continuous facial grimaces and periodically twisting her trunk and her arms in choreoathetoid movements."

Epilepsy and convulsive disorders affect between 1 and 2% of the population, and can occur at virtually any age. Epileptic seizures, which are caused by abnormal electrical activity in the brain, can range from a brief lapse of attention to a prolonged loss of consciousness. One of the most common is the so-called grand mal seizure. There is a loss of muscle control, and a cry is often produced as the individual falls to the floor. After a series of rhythmic jerking contractions of the arms and legs, during which time incontinence and tongue biting may occur, the patient gradually regains consciousness. Headache and drowsiness are common afterward, and the individual may not recover fully for several days.

Such seizures can develop following a diminution in the inhibitory activity of a natural brain chemical called gamma-aminobutyric acid (GABA). Doctors at Beth Israel–Deaconess Medical Center in Boston have recently injected fetal pig cells into the brain of a middle-aged man with severe epilepsy. The researchers hope the pig brain cells will form connections with the patient's own brain cells and secrete enough GABA to prevent the seizures. This medical team plans to transplant pig cells into as many as seven more epileptic patients during the next year or two.

Spinal cord diseases or injury

For years, surgeons have dreamed of restoring movement to lifeless limbs caused by spinal cord injury or disease. Actor Christopher Reeve, who was paralyzed following a horse riding accident, is one of 8,000 new spinal cord injury patients in the United States each year. The National Spinal Cord Injury Association estimates that 200,000 U.S. citizens have suffered some form of spinal cord injury. The recent attempt by surgeons in Gainesville, Florida, to treat a patient with a rare crippling spinal cord disease, known as syringomyelia, with human fetal nerve cells may be the beginning of a new era in this field. It has long been maintained that fibers in the adult central nervous system cannot regenerate. However, several studies in animals have shown that fetal cell transplants can improve function after spinal cord injury. Recently, Ying Li and his associates at the National Institute for Medical Research in the United Kingdom found that stem cells derived from adult animals could also be used to treat partial division of the spinal cord in rats. Although none of the control animals in the study recovered after injury to the spinal cord, four of the seven transplanted animals recovered a forepaw-reaching function. In these animals, the transplanted cells formed a bridge of tissue across the site of the injury. Although there is clearly a long way to go, scientists are hopeful that in the future the transplantation of porcine cells will help patients recover from spinal cord injury and disease.

A remedy for pain

Thirty-four million Americans (nearly one in five) suffer from some form of chronic pain, which in many cases can be severe enough to destroy normal family life and prevent employment. It has been estimated that chronic pain costs the United States approximately $90 billion each year in medical claims. One of the most feared forms of pain is cancer-related. Two-thirds of all patients with advanced cancer suffer significant discomfort which, despite enormous medical advances, may be very resistant to treatment. Cell transplantation offers new hope for these patients.

Chromaffin cells from cows have the ability to secrete natural analgesic

substances, such as opioid peptides. Preliminary clinical trials have been initiated in Europe involving terminal cancer patients suffering from intractable pain who are injected with these cells sequestered inside a tethered
tubular membrane chamber. The chambers are usually implanted into the
lower back in the space that contains the fluid surrounding the spinal cord.
A minimally invasive surgical procedure—"keyhole surgery"—is all that is
required. In two patients who were suffering from facial and neck pain, the
chambers were implanted directly into the brain. The implants have produced no serious complications, and 7 of 10 patients reported less pain and
required measurably smaller doses of narcotics. Pain relief lasting until their
death from cancer—up to five months after receiving the bovine implant—
has been recorded. After death, removal and examination of the chambers
revealed histological and biochemical evidence of bovine cell viability and
function. The FDA has now approved an initial clinical trial in the United
States.

Aid for AIDS ○ ○ ○

David Brudnoy is a well-known author and Boston talk-show host. In 1988,
after a friend suggested that his run-down health was suggestive of something
beyond a lingering cold, he was found to be HIV-positive. "For six years," he
recalls (*Newsweek,* December 2, 1996), "I lumbered along relatively healthy,
keeping my HIV status private." However, in 1994, David developed full-
blown AIDS; his legs swelled and his feet turned purple, his temperature shot
up, and he developed a hacking cough, nausea, and dizziness. "Then, one
night in October, I passed out and was rushed to a hospital, barely escaping
death . . . or so the doctors said. I woke up nine days later." Although he is
now receiving a combination of the new antiretroviral drugs, he still has very
few infection-fighting T lymphocytes—only 71 cells in each milliliter of blood,
whereas healthy people have about 1,200 per milliliter.

David Brudnoy, of course, is not alone. Acquired immune deficiency
syndrome (AIDS) is a global epidemic, with virtually every country in the
world reporting cases. The disease is caused by infection with the human
immunodeficiency viruses (HIV), which leads to a susceptibility to what we
know as "AIDS-defining" diseases, which include serious infections, cancer,
and neurological disease. By 1998, over 30 million people had been infected
with HIV worldwide. One expert estimates that one new person is infected
every 15 seconds.

The main targets for the virus are a subgroup of the white blood cells,
the T lymphocytes, which we have discussed earlier in relation to their role

in the development of organ allograft rejection. Infection with the virus leads to a progressive decline in the number and function of a subset of these cells. This key population controls the induction and/or regulation of virtually the entire immune system.

The possibility of reconstituting the immune system of AIDS patients with bone marrow cells from an animal species whose white blood cells are resistant to the HIV virus would clearly have enormous implications. For reasons that are unclear to scientists, baboons are known to be resistant to infection by HIV and therefore may be a potential source of healthy T cells for patients with AIDS. Based on this reasoning, in December 1995, doctors at San Francisco General Hospital transplanted baboon stem cells—primitive immature cells that can develop into all types of blood cells, including T lymphocytes—into a patient with documented HIV infection. The patient, Jeff Getty (Figure 9.6), claims to be feeling better than he did before the procedure. However, test results suggest that the transplanted baboon cells were destroyed within the first few weeks. Despite being seriously immunodeficient from the HIV infection and receiving low doses of both radiation and chemotherapy, Getty's physicians agree that the therapy they administered probably did not suppress his immune system sufficiently for the AIDS-resistant baboon cells to take root in his body. AIDS-fighting immune cells were therefore not produced. No new trials of this form of therapy appear to be planned at present.

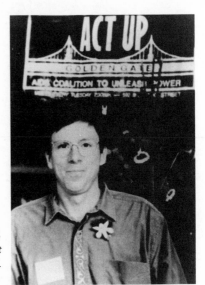

figure 9.6. *In 1995, Jeff Getty, a patient with AIDS, received immune cells from a baboon in an attempt to reinforce his own immune defenses against infection.*

Voronoff's Vision: The Limitless Vista o o o

The pioneering efforts of Serge Voronoff to "rejuvenate" elderly men by the implantation of slices of chimpanzee testes were discussed in Chapter 3. Though his efforts were clearly premature, and indeed subject to criticism and even derision, Voronoff at least perceived the role cell implants could

figure 9.7. *Medical disorders potentially treatable by the transplantation of animal cells.*

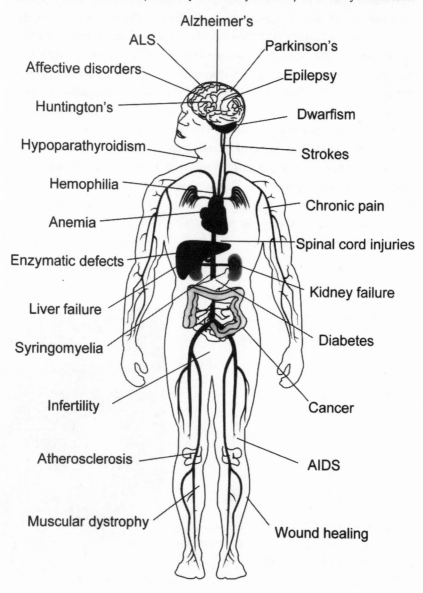

play in replacing functions lost from degeneration of tissues or other causes. For example, French documentary film director Jean Real has drawn attention to the fact that as early as 1913, Voronoff had the vision to transplant the thyroid gland from a chimpanzee into a 14-year-old child in whom the gland was not functioning; his hope was that the transplanted gland would provide the thyroid hormone the child lacked. Whether the transplanted gland ever functioned is extremely unlikely, but four years later the young patient was declared fit for military service!

Much of the work outlined in this chapter has, in fact, been directed toward this aim—the replacement of lost function. With the development of successful xenografting, we might see the dawn of an era of successful cell transplants that provide replacement therapy for a multitude of physiological deficiencies. The potential for culture, cloning, and genetic manipulation of cells adds greatly to the clinical possibilities of this form of therapy.

Researchers are searching for effective therapies for a wide range of disorders that result from tissue loss or cellular dysfunction. These include a variety of diseases in which there is enzyme or hormone deficiency (Figure 9.7). For example, transplantation of cells that produce blood-clotting factors for hemophilia may become possible. Cell transplants that secrete erythropoietin for the treatment of anemia, and growth hormone for the treatment of dwarfism, are potentially possible (Figure 9.8).

Certain rare genetic diseases may also prove amenable to therapy using transplanted porcine cells. In familial hypercholesterolemia, a hereditary defect in the liver results in the individual having a serum cholesterol level that may be as much as 10 to 15 times higher than the safe level in a normal person. As a result of this dangerously high level, even young children in

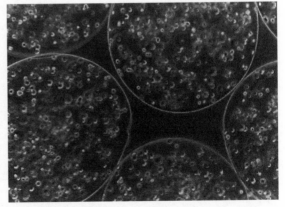

figure 9.8. Encapsulated pig cells genetically engineered to produce human growth hormone. These cells could be transplanted to produce growth hormone in patients afflicted with AIDS or dwarfism. Animal cells can also be engineered to produce other biotherapeutic substances such as clotting factors for hemophilia and nerve growth factors for such diseases as Alzheimer's and Parkinson's.

these families suffer from advanced coronary artery disease. Surgery for an obstructed coronary artery may sometimes be necessary in children under the age of five. A research team at Diacrin has reported that the transplantation of pig hepatocytes into the livers of a certain breed of rabbit that has a very similar disorder led to a reduction in cholesterol levels of 30 to 60%. There is therefore hope that the implantation of normal pig hepatocytes in children susceptible to this disease may prevent the development of coronary artery disease.

As researchers identify new bioactive molecules and expand their understanding of the role specific cells play in human disease processes, the list of deficiencies in which replacement therapy by suitable cell transplants may be possible will undoubtedly continue to grow. If we look into our scientific crystal ball, it may be that many such disorders will be treated not by a pill a day or an injection every three months but by the transplantation of encapsulated cells once every 10 years.

chapter 10

The Discordant Concert

Will the transplanted organ work?

Living out of One's Element ○ ○ ○

Claus Hammer, of the Institute of Surgical Research of the University of Munich in Germany, who is both a qualified physician and a veterinary surgeon, has reviewed many aspects of the topic of whether animal organs are likely to function satisfactorily if transplanted into humans. He has written: "Evolution has set severe obstacles to xenotransplantation. Even in closely-related species combinations, significant differences . . . exist which can profoundly disturb . . . [the] interactions between graft and recipient."

In other words, even if all of the immunological and microbiological hurdles outlined in this book can be overcome successfully, we are faced with the question of whether an animal organ will function normally in the environment of the human body. This involves anatomical considerations (whether the organ is structurally similar to its counterpart in the human) as well as physiological (functional) and biochemical considerations (whether the multitude of enzyme systems, hormones, and so on that function adequately in the organ when in the animal will perform equally successfully when the organ is transferred to the human patient).

Xenotransplanters have therefore set themselves a difficult task. Will they be able to overcome the severe obstacles that have developed over the millennia as a result of evolutionary change?

Hammer points out that of the estimated 2 million animal species on this planet, there are more than 4,000 mammal species, although at least a

147

quarter of these are small rodents. On the basis of their anatomical characteristics, only a handful of species would be suitable as organ donors for humans. With regard to the most likely donor species, namely nonhuman primates and domesticated mammals, anatomical differences are surprisingly small. Baboon or pig hearts and kidneys are structurally very similar to those of humans.

From a functional perspective, there are essentially two questions that need to be answered. First, will a transplanted animal organ continue working normally in the human milieu, or will differences in such conditions as body temperature and the acidity of the blood (pH) adversely affect the organ? For example, enzyme systems can be sensitive to even small differences in pH or temperature. Second, even if the organ works normally, will it fulfill all of the roles of a healthy human organ? The state of our knowledge at present is insufficient to answer either of these questions with confidence, but some aspects of this important subject are of considerable interest.

There may be relatively simple and seemingly minor structural variations between donor animal and human recipient. Let us consider something as basic as the animal's posture. Upright posture is rare in the animal kingdom. Only humans, certain other primates, and kangaroos normally stand and walk (or hop) on two feet. As a result, certain characteristics are rather different in these species from other mammals of comparable size. For example, posture influences blood circulation. Oxygen transport will almost certainly be altered if the lungs or heart from a horizontal donor animal, such as the pig, are transplanted into an upright recipient, such as the human. Whether this difference will be sufficient to affect either the function of the transplanted organ or of the recipient's other organs remains unknown.

If the patient's red blood cells (which carry oxygen) or white blood cells are significantly larger than those of the donor animal, they may have difficulty in traversing the small blood vessels (capillaries) of the grafted organ. Fortunately, red blood cells are generally very elastic and can change their form to squeeze through vessels of small diameter. In contrast, white blood cells vary in size but are relatively rigid, and are more likely to obstruct the capillaries; however, there are far fewer of them in the blood. If either of these cell types occlude the capillaries, then the flow of oxygen and nutrients to the organ's tissues will be reduced. This would almost certainly impair the graft's function. Such an incompatibility would prove a major barrier to successful xenotransplantation, and might prove exceedingly difficult to overcome. For the record, human red blood cells are somewhat larger than their porcine counterparts, and theoretically could block the capillaries of the transplanted organ. However, pig hearts and kidneys have functioned satisfactorily in nonhuman primates for periods of several weeks (until rejection has intervened). It therefore seems unlikely that any difference in size of red or white cells is sufficient to cause prohibitive problems.

Alternatively, the differences between donor and recipient may be functional rather than structural. A large number and diversity of chemical and biological products are required for any organ to perform adequately. Will all of these essential substrates and metabolites be present in the foreign environment of the human recipient to allow normal function of the animal organ? There may be only one enzyme system or hormone that cannot function properly, but this may be a crucial link in the chain that enables the organ to perform its normal duties. For example, the pig's normal temperature is approximately 102.5°F (39°C), 3° to 4°F or so above that of a human (98.6°F; 37°C). The change in temperature may affect certain metabolic activities in the transplanted organ. Enzymes, hormones, and a myriad of biochemical activities may function less efficiently or more slowly at the reduced human temperature.

Sir Roy Calne of the University of Cambridge in the United Kingdom was (in 1970) one of the first to draw attention to what he termed the "milieu interieur" of the recipient. He questioned whether the human body could provide an animal organ with the necessary environmental conditions for good graft function. Our doubts in this respect are greater for organs such as the liver and kidney than for the heart. The heart is a relatively simple muscular pump, whereas the kidney and, in particular, the liver carry out many more complex functions. According to Hammer, the liver—the body's "factory"—produces no fewer than 2,500 different products. The questions raised by Calne still cannot be fully answered, but evidence is slowly beginning to accumulate.

Specific Pig Organs ○ ○ ○

Experimental data indicate that pig hearts and kidneys can function in baboons or monkeys for periods of over two months. This lends encouragement to the view that long-term function of these pig organs will be possible in humans. To date, pig livers have been observed to support life satisfactorily in baboons and monkeys for only three days, and this is clearly an insufficient period of time on which to base a prediction. Experimental experience with transplantation of pig lungs is even more limited, but as the function of these organs is largely mechanical—relating to gas exchange across a membrane— theoretically they should function adequately in a human recipient if the immunological problems can be overcome. However, pig lungs are rapidly and easily damaged by even minor rejection changes or molecular incompatibilities, and it is generally agreed that successful xenotransplantation of this particular organ will be difficult to achieve.

Pigs have been used extensively in research relating to heart function, and data regarding the hemodynamic performance of the pig heart are well documented. There are some minor differences between the action of pig and human hearts. For example, resting heart rate and blood pressure are both somewhat higher in the pig than in a human of corresponding size. Still, the similarities between the two are many. The evidence would appear to indicate that the pig heart will function satisfactorily in a human, both at rest and during exercise, if factors not directly related to the heart (such as the body temperature and acidity of the blood) do not influence the outcome.

There is, however, one potential, though perhaps minor, problem in this respect. Although wild pigs are excellent runners, modern domesticated pigs lead extremely inactive, sedentary lives. Being reared in confined spaces, they take virtually no exercise, and certainly no sustained exercise, through which they might develop some cardiovascular conditioning. They are like human couch potatoes; although healthy, they cannot be considered fit in the generally accepted sense. This lack of fitness may have a detrimental effect on the performance of the pig's heart, particularly after it has been transplanted into a human recipient and is expected to support an active, mobile subject.

Comparative studies have been carried out by a research group headed by Harvard heart surgeons Gus Vlahakes and Joren Madsen. The results indicate that when the heart is stressed to increase its workload (as would occur during exercise), the output of the average pig heart increases to a lesser degree than its human counterpart of similar size. Although it may seem mildly ridiculous, it is not inconceivable that pigs being reared as donors of hearts for humans will have to be regularly exercised—perhaps on a treadmill—in order to improve their conditioning before transplantation. Alternatively, of course, if the heart can support the patient successfully through the transplant operation, it can be conditioned later as the patient steadily increases his/her exercise program during rehabilitation. Nevertheless, it would clearly be best to start out with a porcine athlete's heart at the time of the transplant.

Speculation over the ability of other pig organs—kidney, pancreas, and liver—to function adequately in humans was put forward some years ago by former Harvard transplant surgeon Robert Kirkman. In 1989 he concluded that as kidney size, anatomical structure, and metabolic and regulatory parameters are all similar between pigs and humans, there is no evidence to suggest that pig kidneys will not work adequately in humans. The accuracy of Kirkman's predictions is slowly being supported by experiments carried out by the British biotechnology company, Imutran, headed by University of Cambridge transplant surgeon Peter Friend. Friend's group has transplanted kidneys from pigs transgenic for the human complement regulatory protein, decay accelerating factor (DAF), into monkeys. Some of these kidneys have survived without rejection for periods approaching three months, sustaining near-normal function throughout most of this time. In only one or two respects has there been evidence of inadequate or abnormal function. For example, the electrolyte balance changes with time (Table 10.1). Whereas sodium and potassium remain within the normal human range, calcium increases and phosphate disappears almost completely. These changes, the exact cause of which remains uncertain, could have far-reaching effects on the body's activity if left uncontrolled.

Pig livers have been used relatively successfully in cross-circulation systems in patients with fulminant liver failure to provide temporary life-sustaining support and have therefore been demonstrated to perform at least some of the functions necessary to support human life. However, it is unlikely that *all* of the enzymes and hormones of the pig liver will function with equal efficiency in human recipients. Nevertheless, for those of us who enjoy an occasional glass of wine—or even a fairly frequent one—Hammer reports what can only be considered good news: the pig liver metabolizes alcohol at

table 10.1

Comparison of Serum Electrolyte Levels (in mMol/L) in Humans and Pigs

		Range
Sodium	Human	140 — 160
	Pig	135 — 144
Potassium	Human	40 — 50
	Pig	36 — 48
Calcium	Human	2.4 — 3.0
	Pig	2.2 — 2.5
Phosphate	Human	5.0 — 8.3
	Pig	2.6 — 4.5
Chloride	Human	102 — 106
	Pig	97 — 108

Data provided by Claus Hammer.

a faster rate than its human counterpart. Transplantation of a pig liver into a human might also cause complex immunological problems. Complement, which is activated by human antibodies to cause the destruction of a transplanted pig organ, is manufactured in the liver. Removal of a diseased human liver will therefore remove the source of human complement. This would seem to be an advantage, as there would no longer be any human complement to destroy the pig liver that will replace its human counterpart. Furthermore, the transplanted pig liver will produce pig complement, which is very inefficient in damaging pig tissues; this would improve the chances of survival of the pig liver. But will the pig complement be injurious to all of the other organs in the patient's body—the human tissues? These tissues are protected by complement regulatory proteins that are effective against human complement, but may be far less effective against pig complement. We do not know the answer to this conundrum.

Pig and human insulins differ in molecular structure by only one amino acid. Pig insulin has been used to control glucose levels in diabetic patients for over 70 years. Since the regulation of insulin secretion in the pig is very similar to that in humans, pig pancreatic islet cells will probably function successfully after transplantation. Humans, however, have a slightly higher normal blood glucose level than pigs. Although the pig islets may adapt to this need, it is conceivable that the stimulus provided by this higher glucose level could induce the pig islets to overproduce insulin and consequently exhaust themselves. As yet, we have no experimental experience to suggest whether this problem will arise.

Let us examine just one or two of the myriad of factors that comparative physiologist Claus Hammer has pointed out may influence the ability of an organ from one species to successfully replace that of another.

The Effect of Evolution ○ ○ ○

Biochemical data provide a more precise classification of various animal species than do structural characteristics, and so they allow a judgment to be made regarding the metabolic compatibility between two species. For example, albumin is a protein present in large quantities in the blood. Albumin is made up of a sequence of amino acids that is known to change at a similar rate in different species over a given period of evolutionary time. The more recent the common ancestor that the two species share, the closer will be the amino acid sequences. The differences in albumins between species help to determine the degree and timing of evolutionary change—the so-called

immunological clock. Table 10.2 shows the much greater evolutionary difference between humans (with a score of 1) and pigs (with a relative score
of >35) than between humans and the higher nonhuman primates (with
relative scores of <3). Using albumin as an indicator, therefore, the very
considerable differences between humans and pigs that have resulted from
evolutionary change are made abundantly clear. Whether they are sufficient
to wreck our long-term plans for xenotransplantation remains uncertain.

A difference in albumin is important in itself, not just as a marker of
evolutionary change. Albumin is a major carrier molecule, for example, of
cholesterol, bilirubin, and steroid hormones. The albumins of pig and human
are so different in molecular structure and chemical behavior that Hammer
questions whether a compatible carrier function can be expected.

table 10.2

*Comparison of the Evolutionary Relationship Between
Certain Primate and Nonprimate Species*

Species	Index of Dissimilarity*
Primates	
Humans and apes	
Human	1.0
Chimpanzee	1.14
Gorilla	1.09
Orangutan	1.22
Gibbon	1.28–1.30
Old World monkeys	2.23–2.65
New World monkeys	2.7–5.0
Prosimians (e.g., lemur)	8.6–18
Nonprimates	
Bull	32
Pig	>35

Adapted from the work of V. M. Sarich. In: *Perspectives on Human
Evolution*, S. L. Washburn and P. C. Jay (eds.). New York: Holt,
Rinehard and Winston, 1968.

*Based on reactivity in the microcomplement fixation test to hu-
man serum albumin. The greater the discrepancy from 1.0, the
more distant is the evolutionary relationship with humans.

The Molecular "Concert" ○ ○ ○

As indicated by the immunological clock, the physiological parameters of closely related species, such as humans and apes, are almost identical. Once we attempt to cross the barrier of a zoological family, however, major differences may arise. Many basic metabolic characteristics are common to all mammals, and differ only in detail. However, they are dependent on coordinated contact between the cells that make up the organs of the body. Secreted messenger molecules of one cell that carry a chemical message to another cell must be compatible with the receptor on the other cell. Hammer has described the interactions of these myriad signal molecules and their targets as a "concert": all have to play together if the music is to be enjoyed. Some idea of the complexity of this concert and of how organ xenotransplantation might affect its smooth functioning can be gleaned from the following brief outline.

Most signal molecules are proteins that are specific to one species, such as the pig, and this fact alone may cause problems after xenotransplantation. However, because of the potent action of these messenger molecules, once they have fulfilled their function they have to be destroyed. This is carried out by inhibitor molecules that may also be species-specific. To add to the complexity, different cells have different receptors and may therefore respond differently to the same signal. Furthermore, some signal molecules, such as many in the brain, affect only the adjacent cell, while others, such as hormones, circulate in the bloodstream and influence cells throughout the body. Many of these latter molecules require transport molecules to take them where needed; these are also frequently species-specific.

The physiological and biochemical variations between species may include discrepancies with regard to hemoglobin, blood viscosity, blood groups, enzyme and hormone functions, and blood coagulation. Let us consider one brief example: hormones. Some hormones produced by the liver are likely to work well after xenotransplantation. Steroid hormones, for example, function as sexual hormones or are involved in the regulation of carbohydrate and mineral metabolism. Steroids seem to be biologically similar in all mammals, though they are present in different concentrations in different species. In contrast, hormones constructed of peptides, which perform many essential functions in the body, differ widely from species to species. Their fast action is regulated by similarly fast inhibitors, which are in most cases also species-specific. In addition, there is a complex chain of intermediate molecules and enzymes, any or all of which may differ between two given species. These intermediaries have to be integrated into the sequence to effect a satisfactory result. One disparate factor could disrupt the entire sequence of events.

It is, of course, feasible to breed transgenic pigs that produce a human enzyme or hormone. If only one critical incompatibility were identified, then this approach would resolve the problem. However, if several incompatibilities—or even hundreds—are found to be important, then this approach may prove extremely difficult or even impossible.

Because of the above considerations (and others), Claus Hammer remains concerned that pig organs may function inadequately in the human environment. The following are a few of the many potential problems he has raised.

Cholesterol: too high or too low?

The concentration of serum cholesterol, which is produced by the liver and is necessary for the building of cells, is on average approximately 200 mg/100 ml in humans, but in pigs is much lower at 45 mg/100 ml. Although this difference may be partly due to differences in diet, it is conceivable that the transplantation of a pig liver into a patient with a dangerously high blood cholesterol may lead to a dramatic fall in the level, with a concomitant beneficial effect. However, a very low cholesterol level may be inadequate, as cholesterol plays an important role in developing and maintaining the structure of the human body's cells. (An illustration of this type of metabolic difference comes from experience with the transplantation of baboon livers into two patients at the University of Pittsburgh in 1992 and 1993. The uric acid level in baboons is much lower than in humans. After the transplant, both patients recorded very low levels of uric acid.) It could be that a pig heart or kidney, programmed to function in a low-cholesterol environment, might be particularly susceptible to atherosclerosis when forced to function in a human's high-cholesterol environment.

To clot or to bleed?

Most of the proteins that are involved in clotting (coagulation) of the blood are manufactured in the liver. If a liver is transplanted across a species barrier, then the recipient will be provided with hemostatic proteins (those involved in clotting) from the donor species. Some of these factors are found at much higher levels in the pig than in the human, whereas others are at lower levels. Some pig factors clearly carry out their usual role in humans. For example, porcine Factor VIII has been used to successfully treat hemophilia in humans. But other factors have been shown to be incompatible between pig and human. Such molecular differences could decrease the ability of the blood to clot, leading to spontaneous or prolonged bleeding. Alternatively, they could increase it, leading to thrombosis, in which spontaneous clotting could occlude blood vessels, interrupting the blood supply to certain areas or organs.

Growth hormone: will it still work?

The function of growth hormone is not only to control body and organ growth, but also to influence the utilization of proteins, carbohydrates, and fats. The structures of growth hormones differ between primates in their amino acid sequence by only 2%, but the difference between human and pig is about 19%. Further evidence of this incompatibility is provided by the fact that the growth hormone of one species will not always function as anticipated on an organ of another species.

For example, transgenic mice carrying bovine (cow) or porcine (pig) growth hormone genes develop into giant mice. The foreign growth hormone clearly works, but there is no check on its activity by a matching inhibitor, with a resultant overproduction of the hormone. This not only leads to large body size but may have many detrimental effects, such as kidney damage. In contrast, bovine growth hormone has no effect on growth in humans. This raises the important question of whether a transplanted adult (full-size) animal organ would grow satisfactorily in a human who is not yet full-grown. Conversely, under the influence of human growth hormone, would a transplanted animal organ continue to grow and become a giant organ?

Most pigs will grow to an extremely large size if allowed to do so—sometimes in excess of 450 kg (approximately 1,000 lb). Questions have therefore been raised as to whether a xenografted pig organ will eventually grow too large for the human body in which it has been placed. Will the heart from a young 80-kg (176-lb) pig stop growing in an adult human of equal size? Or will it continue to grow as if it were still in a pig that will eventually weigh 450 kg? The answer is uncertain, but may depend on whether growth of the pig organ is stimulated only by pig growth hormone or can be influenced by human growth hormone.

As the pig heart will no longer be in a pig body, it should theoretically no longer be stimulated by pig growth hormone unless the pig organ has some inbuilt mechanism that continues to stimulate it to grow. Even if a pig organ could be stimulated to grow by the presence of human growth hormone, the production of human growth hormone in the adult human recipient should be reduced, as he or she has finished growing. In theory, therefore, neither pig growth hormone nor human growth hormone should stimulate the pig heart to grow further.

However, early observations from pig kidney transplants in monkeys performed by the Imutran group in the United Kingdom provided some intriguing food for thought. It initially appeared that kidneys from infant pigs (of less than 6 weeks of age and weighing approximately 5 kg) when transplanted into adult monkeys of similar weight (5 to 8 kg) continued to grow quickly, as if they were still in a rapidly growing piglet. Within two months, some of the kidneys had almost doubled in size, whereas the monkey's weight remained unchanged. This suggested that the pig kidney was growing even in the absence of high levels of growth hormone (and certainly in the absence of pig growth hormone). Longer-term observations by this group now suggest that some of this increase in kidney size may be related to rejection, when fluid and cells collect in the graft, but this is unlikely to fully explain the rapid and considerable enlargement that has been observed.

If growth of an organ were to continue, eventually its sheer bulk would become a problem. Constriction of a large pig heart, for example, in the chest of a small human patient might well prevent the heart from beating effectively. One way of ensuring that this does not occur would be to use a donor pig from a breed that does not grow excessively large. There are several breeds of miniature swine that weigh between 90 and 110 kg (200–250 lb) at full maturity. A heart implanted in an adult human patient from a weight-matched miniature breed would not be expected to grow much larger.

If the transplanted pig organ proved insensitive to human growth hormone, however, other problems would arise. Consider, for example, a heart from an infant pig that does not respond to human growth hormone. If it is transplanted into an infant human, both pig and infant weighing, say, 2.5 kg (5.5 lb), the pig heart will basically remain the same size as when it was transplanted. The child, however, will steadily grow, and within a very few years the small heart will no longer be able to supply the needs of the much larger body. Retransplantation with a larger pig heart will be the only solution. And further transplants will be required every few years until the child reaches full adult size. This is not a pleasant prospect, as retransplant operations generally become more difficult and are associated with a higher risk on each occasion.

Aging of tissues

Pigs have a natural life span of about 15 to 20 years, although they are rarely allowed to reach it. Will the pig organ begin to deteriorate from the aging process as it approaches this point? Or will it take on the aging characteristics of its human host? An organ transplanted into a young adult ideally should function for 40 to 50 years or so. If it begins to age and fail after only 15 years, it would, of course, be necessary to replace it with another pig organ. A few organs taken from elderly human donors have continued to function in younger human recipients long after the donors would have died from natural causes. However, the number of such documented cases is relatively small, and this is not an adequate analogy to pig-to-human transplants.

Erythropoietin and red blood cell production

Erythropoietin is a protein manufactured in the kidneys that stimulates production of red blood cells. Without erythropoietin, the red blood cells are not replaced at the correct rate and the patient becomes anemic. Anemia is associated with many symptoms, not least a lack of energy and tiredness. If untreated, it can eventually lead to death.

If a pig kidney is transplanted into a human or other primate (and the recipient's own kidneys are removed), the recipient would rely on pig erythropoietin for his or her needs. Unfortunately, evidence from both the laboratory of Patrick Aebischer, of the University of Lausanne, in Switzerland, and from the Imutran group indicates that erythropoietin of one species may not always function adequately in another. Pig erythropoietin does not appear to function adequately in primates. Fortunately, as human erythropoietin can be made by recombinant techniques, the recipient of the pig kidney can receive regular injections as replacement therapy. In the Imutran monkeys transplanted with pig kidneys, human recombinant erythropoietin appears to prevent them from becoming anemic.

The situation, however, may be more complex than it might seem. There is evidence from Aebischer's laboratory that one species may make antibodies against erythropoietin of another species. For example, if humans made antibodies against erythropoietin produced by a transplanted pig kidney, these antibodies would cause destruction of the pig erythropoietin. Given that the human body cannot utilize the pig erythropoietin, this may at first glance seem not to matter. Aebischer's experimental data, however, indicate that the antibodies against the foreign erythropoietin may also destroy the recombinant human erythropoietin that is being administered to stimulate production of red blood cells. The result would be that the recipient of the organ would remain without erythropoietin of any sort, and would therefore remain chronically anemic.

If this happened to the human recipient of a pig kidney, the patient may require frequent and regular blood transfusions. The benefits of the pig kidney transplant, which might otherwise be functioning well, would be greatly undermined. Fortunately, Aebischer's fears may be unfounded. The Imutran group has observed that, although erythropoietin from a transplanted pig kidney does not appear to work in recipient monkeys, the (heavily immunosuppressed) monkeys do not make antibodies against the pig erythropoietin. Nor do they make antibodies against the human recombinant erythropoietin with which they are successfully treated. If they were not heavily immunosuppressed, however, they might well make antibodies against pig erythropoietin that cross-react with the human recombinant form.

If time confirms that human recombinant erythropoietin does indeed work in immunosuppressed baboons (or humans) with transplanted pig kidneys, then the ultimate solution might be to use genetic engineering techniques to incorporate the human gene for erythropoietin into the pig kidney. The kidney would therefore produce both pig and human erythropoietin.

The risk that the human recipient may make antibodies against *any* protein produced by a transplanted pig organ—for example, any of the hundreds that would be manufactured by a transplanted liver—and thus destroy that protein may prove to be one of the major limiting factors to successful xenotransplantation. It may certainly prevent successful liver transplantation.

A New Science: Xenoincompatibility o o o

The structure and function of the products of a perfectly functioning animal organ in a human clearly have not yet been investigated. However, once scientists achieve long-term survival of such grafts, their function can be properly assessed. This will open up a whole new area of medicine and biology, namely, the incompatibility of biochemical systems. Extensive investigation and modification will undoubtedly be required if xenotransplantation is to be as successful as we hope and intend. It is conceivable that some incompatibilities may prove to be major limiting factors in the success of xenotransplantation until the problems have been resolved. Indeed, Claus Hammer, the guru in this field, remains relatively pessimistic on this point.

chapter 11

The Hottest Zone

The fear of an AIDS-like epidemic

The Ever-Present Fear ○ ○ ○

The young man is barely conscious—fortunately so, for his condition is, by any standards, pitiable. Despite the cold-water-soaked towels that are laid across and around his body, he sweats profusely, and his jaundiced skin is seemingly on fire to the touch. His lethargy is punctuated by periods in which he rolls around in a state of delirium. Blood oozes from every body orifice. When he coughs, he brings up blood; when he vomits, his vomitus is heavily bloodstained. Five days ago he had been seemingly well, except for a head-ache and a chill. Today will be his last day in this world; he will be dead by midnight, an event that will be accompanied by much wailing by his ex-tended family, who wait outside in the mission hospital's little lobby.

The nurses are doing their best, as is the Belgian doctor who mans this outpost in the heart of Central Africa, but they are helpless in the face of one of the world's most efficient killers—the Ebola virus. Even if the patient were at one of the great teaching hospitals of Boston or London, however, his case would be equally hopeless. There is no known cure for Ebola fever, and how it spreads remains a mystery. Once Ebola infects you, the chances are 9 to 1 that you will not see out the week. Ebola is one of a group of viruses that cause infectious hemorrhagic fever, in which the body loses its ability to prevent bleeding from all of its membranes, and the patient dies a very un-pleasant death.

Other viruses in this group include the Marburg virus, so named because it killed a number of citizens of that German town in 1967 who became infected by handling tissues from wild African green monkeys captured in Uganda. There are at least 15 other viruses that cause this condition, several in Africa, such as the less violent Rift Valley fever (which is estimated to infect up to 100,000 people annually) and Lassa fever. The Crimean-Congo hemorrhagic fever kills 30 to 50% of those it infects, not only in Africa, but also in parts of Asia and Europe.

But in this day and age of air transportation, such diseases are no longer confined to isolated areas of the world such as central Africa or Asia. The Marburg outbreak is witness to that, and there have been other sporadic outbreaks before and since. What if just one infected patient should board a plane and mingle, not only with the other passengers, but with the inhabitants at the point of debarkation? What was of concern only in distant Congo yesterday could become a nightmare to the public health authorities in New York today. Fortunately, most of these outbreaks to date have remained localized. Since these viruses cause such obvious illness in the victims they infect, the outbreaks were controlled—and quickly died down—once sensible steps were taken to prevent further spread.

There are diagnostic tests available that can identify the viruses that we know can cause such hemorrhagic fevers. But at the Centers for Disease Control and Prevention (CDC) in Atlanta, Georgia, one of the world's great compositories of information on such diseases, virologists receive a handful or so specimens of blood and tissues each year in which the infecting microorganism—probably a virus—cannot be identified by any of the tests available. These samples, sent from various countries around the world, are from patients who have died of similar diseases. In other words, the disease may have been caused by a totally new virus, hitherto unknown even to the world's greatest experts. The human hold on the world clearly remains tenuous when there are unknown, lethal viruses demanding of our attention every few months. The original source of the virus—or at least the carrier— is sometimes suspected of being a wild animal, perhaps a monkey, although it is rarely possible to confirm this. The virus is possibly carried from one host to another by a tick, mosquito, or rodent.

With more insidious viruses, widespread, even global spread can take place before the seriousness of the condition has been recognized. The AIDS pandemic, accounting to date for 12 million deaths worldwide with 250,000 new infections each month, is a prime example. There is compelling evidence that it was spread to humans from African nonhuman primate species. Data "suggest that the HIV-2 epidemic in West Africa," wrote Louisa Chapman and her colleagues at the CDC, the Scripps Research Institute, and the U.S.

Food and Drug Administration (*New England Journal of Medicine*, November 30, 1995), "began with the transmission of SIV [simian immunodeficiency virus] from a sooty mangabey [monkey] into a human, with subsequent transmission among humans. In Central Africa, the cross-species transmission of SIV from a different species of primate, probably the chimpanzee, appears to have resulted in the HIV-1 pandemic." Spread of the viruses took place across continents over a number of years before the nature of the disease they caused was identified. This delay in recognition was simply because the disease was not rapidly fatal but took some years of incubation before it became symptomatic in the infected person.

Transplanting a Microbe o o o

Could a disease equally as devastating as AIDS be transmitted by means of an animal donor organ to a transplant patient? This is an important question to the patient about to undergo xenotransplantation. Of much greater importance from the public health view, however, is whether an infected patient could then transfer the infectious organism—probably a virus—to those with whom he or she comes into contact. As many viruses are spread through the air and breathed in by the victim, this would presumably include the medical and hospital staff as well as family and friends. Another virus might spread in a different way, and so potential victims might include, say, all of an infected person's sexual contacts.

Infection transferred with a donor organ is not a new phenomenon. There is a significant risk of transferring an infectious agent when a human organ is transplanted, and numerous cases have been documented. Indeed, viral agents, such as cytomegalovirus and Epstein-Barr virus, are very commonly transferred. Other organisms, such as parasites and bacteria, can also be a problem.

These transferred microbes are of particular risk to an organ transplant patient because he or she will receive heavy immunosuppressive drug therapy, seriously affecting his or her natural resistance to infection. Furthermore, certain viruses are known to lead to cancerous conditions in the patient, and others may possibly increase the severity of rejection episodes affecting the grafted organ. (It is quite likely that viruses transferred with a pig organ would have the same effects.) When the organism is a virus, such as the hepatitis viruses (which cause liver disease), there is a risk of subsequent spread from the organ transplant recipient to those in close contact. Even HIV has been transferred with an organ transplant.

The Risk of Cross-Species Infection ∘ ∘ ∘

The transfer of infection from animals to humans is certainly recognized, but is usually based on direct animal-to-human physical contact. Such is the case with diseases such as anthrax and rabies. However, some infections, once spread from the original animal source, can disseminate through the human population. We have already mentioned this in relation to AIDS. The perception that this risk is much higher if nonhuman primates are used as the organ donors has been one of the major reasons why these species are no longer being considered seriously for this role. However, the risks associated with use of the pig are not negligible.

The great influenza pandemic of 1918 provides a dramatic example. There is evidence that influenza viruses reside harmlessly in birds and are passed into pigs, usually from ducks or other nearby waterfowl. Once infected, the immune system of the pig attacks the virus. But mutant strains of the virus may survive. Such mutations in the virus's genetic makeup may have made the 1918 virus much more virulent when it was transferred from pigs into people. The result was devastating. The new virus spread far and fast, carried rapidly around the world within months, in part by troops mobilized for the First World War. The epidemic swept not only the United States and Europe, but virtually every region of the world—southern Africa, Siberia, even the most remote islands of the Pacific. Within a year, it had killed an estimated 20 million to 40 million people, including 675,000 in the United States alone (ten times more than the nation lost in World War I, and almost twice the total number of U.S. deaths caused by AIDS to date). According to Jeffrey Taubenberger, a member of the scientific team that provided the first direct genetic evidence that the 1918 flu virus came into humans from pigs, "It was really an unbelievable nightmare. There was a very high death rate, and a shortage of morticians, coffins, and gravediggers" (*Boston Globe*, March 21, 1997).

The 1918 experience has not been the only flu pandemic. Indeed, worldwide epidemics seem to occur every 20 to 50 years, with minor local outbreaks in between. Major pandemics were documented as far back as 1627, with what was called the "English sweat." Many experts feared that the 1997 outbreak in Hong Kong heralded a pandemic that might be even more dangerous than the 1918 experience. The Hong Kong outbreak appeared to be related to direct transfer of a virus from chickens into humans, bypassing the porcine middleman. This outbreak was viewed so seriously by the Hong Kong health authorities that they ordered the slaughter of no less than 1.25 million chickens.

With the exception of influenza, it could be argued that the risk of infection from pigs to humans is small. Serious outbreaks of other infections in pigs do occur, however, sometimes caused by a previously unrecognized virus, as evidenced by the 1999 Nipah virus epidemic in Malaysia. More than 100 pig farmers and other close contacts died, necessitating the Malaysian military to shoot 2 million pigs in an effort to eradicate the disease. Nevertheless, with these occasional exceptions, we have bred, fed, lived with, eaten, and slaughtered pigs for generations, and the incidence of pig-derived zoonoses in humans is small. Pig farmers, slaughterers, or butchers, who most frequently expose themselves to pig tissue through cuts on their hands, do not appear to suffer from any terrible, intractable diseases as a result of this exposure. The skin from pigs has been applied as temporary cover in many patients with extensive burns; no serious infections appear to have been transferred. Perhaps we therefore do not need to be too concerned about the risk of infection from xenotransplantation.

The direct implantation of an animal organ into a human subject, however, opens up a new dimension in the possible transfer of microbes between two species. Transfer no longer depends on direct physical contact between an infected animal and a human or, alternatively, on some vector (such as an insect) to transfer the microbe from the animal to the human. In xenotransplantation, the animal organ will be placed permanently within the human body, which may well provide ideal conditions for reproduction and growth of any microorganisms transferred with it. The transplanted organ, oxygenated and nourished by the surrounding human tissues, may act as a perfect culture medium for multiplication of the microorganisms, possibly allowing their dispersal throughout the entire human body. This is a method of transfer that medical science has not had to consider previously. To differentiate an infection transferred by xenotransplantation from a run-of-the-mill zoonosis, Harvard physician Jay Fishman and other microbiologists have suggested the names "xenozoonosis" or "xenosis."

Fishman and other infectious-disease experts have pointed out that the problems associated with infection may be greater following xenotransplantation than after allotransplantation for a number of reasons. First, the organisms transferred from the pig may not be identifiable by routine laboratory tests. Second, the way in which the infection presents in the patient may differ from the traditional clinical symptoms and signs of infection with which transplant physicians have become accustomed. The infection may therefore go unrecognized. Third, the infecting microbe might undergo changes in biological behavior or mutational adaptation or acquire new pieces of genetic material (DNA) within the human host. For example, prolonged infection with the influenza virus in an immunocompromised host can lead to mutation of the virus. This may lead to the virus being more (or less) virulent. Finally, having never been exposed to the porcine organism or any related organism previously, the patient may have no preexisting immunity to the pathogen, which may therefore multiply unimpeded.

There are many examples in the medical literature of microbes that have proven lethal when introduced into a group who have no natural resistance to the organism. One of the classic examples is the spread of smallpox, introduced by European sailors and settlers, in North America. Smallpox killed thousands of Native Americans, who had not been exposed to this virus previously and had thus developed no resistance to it. This might be the case if a novel pig virus were transferred to humans.

Furthermore, some of the steps we may take to prevent rejection of a transplanted pig organ might actually increase the risk of infection. The patient's anti-Gal antibodies, for example, are part of the human defense against certain bacteria, viruses and parasites. Normally, by binding to Gal molecules on the surface of these microbes, complement is activated and the microbe is destroyed. Removal of these antibodies from the patient to prevent graft rejection, particularly for a prolonged period of time, might increase his or her susceptibility to certain infections. As a second example, some of the human complement-regulatory proteins, such as membrane cofactor protein (MCP) and decay accelerating factor (DAF), are themselves receptors for certain viruses and bacteria. The infectiousness of a virus may be increased up to a millionfold by the presence of such a receptor. A pig organ transgenic for one or more of these human proteins may be particularly susceptible to infection by a specific microorganism.

We shall therefore have to be extremely thorough in eradicating microbes from the donor animal. The presence of an infection within the transplanted organ could damage the organ, even if the infection were not passed on to the patient. Furthermore, even if a microbe is known *not* to cause disease in the donor pig, it will have to be excluded from the pig because there is no guarantee that it will not cause disease in the human recipient.

There are several examples of viruses carried by one animal species, without any signs of ill health, that can be rapidly fatal when transferred to another species. The herpes B virus, for example, is commonly found in certain species of monkey, where it seemingly results in no problems, but when transferred to humans, it can quickly lead to death. This was brought home with great impact at the end of 1997 by the tragic death of a young woman at a primate center in Atlanta, Georgia. Although only splashed in the eye with fluid from a monkey she was carrying in a cage, she died within days from an unrecognized herpes B viral infection.

In contrast, some viruses that cause serious infection in humans may not infect the donor animal species. For example, human hepatitis B or HIV-1 infections do not appear to infect baboons. Nor do those two viruses or the herpes viruses, which include the human cytomegalovirus (CMV), appear to infect pigs. The existence of resistance to human viruses by the transplanted animal organ or, conversely, resistance to animal viruses by the human recipient would prove a bonus for xenotransplantation over allotransplantation.

There may therefore be some advantages in using pigs rather than human donors. For example, the transfer of human CMV from a human cadaveric donor to the organ recipient is a common occurrence, and the resulting CMV infection can lead to serious illness and even death of the transplant patient. Human resistance to pig CMV may protect the organ recipient. Nevertheless, it is much more likely that steps will be taken to ensure that the pig donor is totally free of CMV.

It should be easy to ensure that well-known disease-causing microbes are not present in the donor pig. Nevertheless, Frederick Murphy, a leading virologist at the University of California at Davis, estimates that there are already about 4,000 known virus species, with as many as 30,000 strains and variants that infect humans, animals, plants, invertebrates, and other microorganisms. It is inconceivable that there are not many more out there waiting to be discovered, and so there may be other organisms present in animal tissues that may cause disease if transferred by xenotransplantation to humans. The risk of the unknown will always remain. It is the risk that society will have to consider even after every effort has been made to eradicate or minimize the risk of infection from *known* microbes. During the Institute of Medicine workshop held in Washington, DC, in 1995, the point was made repeatedly that society will be obliged to choose between two potential types of harm—that to people who suffer from illness potentially treatable by xenografts, and that to the general population, who might potentially suffer from infectious diseases let loose by xenotransplantation.

Making the Donor Animal Safe ○ ○ ○

How can the risk of the transfer of infection from donor pig to human recipient be minimized? The initial breeding herd will be delivered by caesarean section, which allows them to avoid a number of microbial agents that could infect them as they pass down the birth canal of the sow. The piglets will be transferred immediately into isolators, where they will be environmentally isolated for two weeks from the outside world. Air entering the isolator will be filtered, and all food will be sterilized. The animals will need to be hand-reared during this period, but the handler will not be allowed direct contact with them. The handler will tend to the growing piglets by inserting his or her hands into rubber gloves built into the walls of the isolator. These precautions ensure that the pigs remain germ-free and infection-free throughout this period of isolation.

(Although it is possible to maintain a pig under such gnotobiotic conditions for several months, it is a major undertaking. Because of their rapid growth, their maintenance in isolators presents technical and logistic difficulties.) After two weeks, therefore, the breeding herd will be transferred to a clean, if not totally microbe-free, environment for the remainder of their lives. Once out of the isolator, the pigs are exposed to environmental microbes, and their gastrointestinal tracts become colonized by many bacteria and viruses, even though these rarely cause any ill health. Indeed, some of these organisms may be beneficial to the health of the herd. Subsequent litters—those that will provide the actual donor organs—will not be housed in isolators. This would be enormously time-consuming and immensely expensive, and would increase the cost of donor organs markedly. They will, however, be housed in an extremely clean environment.

In order to prevent the pigs from being exposed to serious infectious agents, the building in which they are housed will have to be specially designed and expensively maintained. The design will have to ensure that no rodents, birds, or even insects gain access to the pigs, and that all air entering the building is filtered without risk of contamination from any source. The air pressure in the rooms housing the pigs will be maintained at a higher level than the surrounding corridors to ensure that no external air enters except through the filters. Temperature, light, and noise will be highly controlled. All foodstuffs will be sterilized, and the building will be thoroughly cleaned every day.

Perhaps the only risk of infection to these pigs will be from the humans with whom they come into contact. The handlers who care for the pigs, therefore, will have to take numerous precautions to ensure that they do not transfer human infections to the pigs. These precautions will include showering and donning clean clothes on every occasion before they enter the pig area. If the stockmen and women are caring for more than one group of pigs (which will be isolated from other groups to ensure no cross-infection), then they will be required to shower and change clothes between each group. In one such facility in the Netherlands, where pigs are separated this way, some stockmen shower up to 14 times a day in the course of their work. The shower includes washing their hair on each occasion. They change clothes completely and are not even allowed to wear items such as wedding rings or jewelry. All of this will prove a time-consuming and therefore costly procedure. The stockmen will be discouraged from keeping pets at home, will not be allowed contact with other farm animals, and will not be able to work with the pigs if they have any sort of communicable disease themselves, even a head cold.

Once the initial group of pigs is removed from the isolators, they will remain with their cohorts until they are sexually mature (approximately seven months of age). The sows will then be bred by artificial insemination from carefully selected boars. When they themselves deliver their litters, the piglets will remain with them for only a short period of time, probably only five days. After that time, the piglets will be removed from the sows and placed in a separate facility, which will be similarly secure from any biohazards relating to the intrusion of wild animals and/or human infection. The reason for early separation from the sows is that the risk of infection being transferred from sow to piglet increases the longer they stay together. Five days has been found to be long enough for the piglet to gain some immune protection from drinking the sow's milk, but not long enough to allow microorganisms to spread. The sows may also receive certain vaccinations before they give birth, again providing further immunity to the piglets. The piglets will then be raised as a group, but will *always* be isolated from other groups of pigs within the facility.

Transportation of donor animals to distant sites (for example, transplant centers) may compromise the microbiological protection so expensively attained and so closely guarded at the pig facility. Careful attention to the conditions of transportation of the pigs—for example, by shipping them in high-efficiency particulate air (HEPA)-filtered crates—could minimize, but not eliminate, exposure to new diseases during transport. Moreover, when dealing with 200-lb pigs, it would be a complicated and expensive process to crate and ship thousands of them to distant locations every year. Organ procurement and tissue processing facilities will therefore be built at the site where the animals are actually housed and raised. This will have a number of advantages, not only relating to protection from infection. When isolating pancreatic islets, for instance, it is important that the pancreas be processed immediately.

After being anesthetized and scrubbed clean, the donor pigs will be moved into a sterile surgical suite where they will be draped and prepared for surgery. A team of specially trained surgeons will excise the organs—heart, lungs, liver, kidneys, pancreas, and/or other tissues. The organs will be packed in boxes of ice, which will then be rushed by road or air to the awaiting hospitals, where they will be transplanted into patients. Some of the pancreases and livers will be transferred to adjacent rooms for processing into islets or hepatocytes, respectively. Once processed, the isolated cells will either be frozen or maintained in incubators for periods of several weeks to months, at which time they will be transported to hospitals for transplantation into patients.

Monitoring for infectious organisms

Frequent clinical examination of the pigs by the stockmen and veterinarians will indicate whether any disease is present. If one or more pigs begin to show signs of shortness of breath, diarrhea, or weight loss, this would clearly require thorough investigation of the entire group. Furthermore, on each of the three or more occasions on which blood tests are performed—soon after birth, at two months, and at four months—one in approximately 50 piglets will be euthanized as a "sentinel animal" and undergo a complete autopsy to ensure that it is disease free. If any disease is found, then the remaining animals in the group will be investigated for that particular disease. There will be certain diseases that, even if present in only the one sentinel animal, will be considered so serious that culling of the entire group of pigs will be required. There are others that will require some form of treatment of the entire group (e.g., antibiotic therapy), and others that may be considered insignificant in relation to xenotransplantation and therefore require no therapy. Only if the piglets are free of significant infection throughout their lives will they be acceptable as organ donors.

When the pigs are of a size suitable for organ donation (generally at four to eight months), the organs will be excised, at which time further specimens of blood and tissues will be sent for microbiological examination. After the organs have been removed, a full autopsy of each carcass will be performed as a check in the unlikely event that any hitherto unrecognized infection or other disease process is present.

"Mad pig" disease?

There are whole ranges of infectious organisms that have to be absent from the pig if it is to be suitable for organ donation. These include the vast majority of bacteria, excluding those that naturally colonize the intestines—these bacteria will not come into contact with any donor organs—as well as parasites, worms, viruses, and even prions.

Prions (which is short for proteinaceous infectious particles) are extraordinary pathogens that do not fit into any other organism category. They are simply abnormal proteins that appear to lack DNA but which can transfer infection by an unknown mechanism. They cause diseases such as "mad cow" disease (bovine spongiform encephalopathy, or BSE). San Francisco neurologist Stanley Prusiner won the 1997 Nobel Prize for medicine for his identification of this unusual disease form. The recent outbreak of BSE in the United Kingdom has been of great concern because this disease appears to be able to be transferred to humans who have eaten infected beef. Cows were not susceptible to the disease until the practice of feeding them the carcasses of (infected) sheep was initiated, which for many years was considered perfectly safe. (There is currently some concern that lamb and mutton might also be a source of infection to humans.) The outbreak of an unexpected disease in this way has made the authorities in the United Kingdom and elsewhere particularly cautious about xenotransplantation. As prion disease takes many years to cause symptoms, failure to ensure the absence of prions in the donor organs could lead to many hundreds or thousands of xenotransplants being performed before the first symptoms become apparent.

The human version of the disease (Creutzfeldt-Jakob disease, or CJD) is a degenerative disorder that causes injury to the brain, although this may take many years to develop. Initial symptoms include anxiety and delusions, followed not long afterward by a miserable death. (CJD has, by the way, been transferred with a human corneal transplant.) Although not uniformly accepted, there are scientists who believe that the 1996 outbreak of prion disease in humans in Britain might be only the tip of an epidemiological iceberg, and that large numbers of Europeans are unknowingly infected and could ultimately die from the disease.

Fortunately, prion disease has never been identified in pigs, and it appears that they can become infected only if infected tissue is injected directly into their brains. Until relatively recently, pigs were fed animal meat and bone as part of their diet, but unlike cattle, no cases of prion disease have occurred. This practice has now been banned, and animal tissue will certainly not form part of the diet of pigs being specially bred to be donors of organs for humans. It would therefore seem that prion disease can be ruled out as a potential risk for human patients.

The threat within: the endogenous retrovirus

Although it should be possible to exclude all of the significant bacteria, parasites, worms, and prions that might infect donor pigs, it will be more difficult—perhaps impossible—to exclude all of the viruses. The majority of viruses that are known or suspected of causing health problems in pigs or humans can probably be excluded—with one major exception, the endogenous retroviruses. These are essentially viruses and viral particles that have become incorporated into the genome of the cell nucleus and incorporate their genetic blueprint directly into the host cell's DNA. Estimates suggest that between 0.1 and 1% of the DNA that humans presently carry may be made up of such viral particles. Probably all mammalian species have their own specific endogenous retroviruses. At least 30 are known in primates, and 3 have been positively identified in pigs to date. These viral sequences owe their presence in modern animals to past episodes of retroviral infection in their ancestors many thousands of years ago. As the viruses have inserted their genetic code into sperm or egg cells, the offspring of the infected animals retain these viral genes, which are then passed from generation to generation. Over time, most of these vestigial viruses have evolved into noninfectious lengths of DNA and are harmless to their hosts; some, however, have been associated with the development of cancerous conditions. In particular, there is concern that if transferred to another species, they may be capable of causing disease in the other species even though they cause no disease in the native species.

Virologists are worried about what these virus particles would do when the pig cells that contain them are transplanted into human patients. Not only does the transplant offer the pig virus direct access to human cells, but it presents the virus with a uniquely susceptible victim—a patient with an immune system that, in order to prevent rejection of the transplanted organ, may have been severely compromised. Under these circumstances, pig viral particles (proviruses) might be able to give rise to active retroviruses, perhaps causing illness (Figure 11.1). Furthermore, when in the Gal-coated cells of a transplanted pig organ, the retrovirus is susceptible to destruction by the human recipient's anti-Gal antibody response. Once the virus leaves the pig cell and enters a human cell, it is no longer susceptible to this attack. The human defense mechanism has been circumvented. If immunological tolerance to the pig organ has been achieved, the tolerance may extend also to the retrovirus in the transplanted pig tissues. These viruses could thereafter be totally immune to the body's defenses against infection.

It is also conceivable that these pig retroviruses could mutate in human

A

B

C

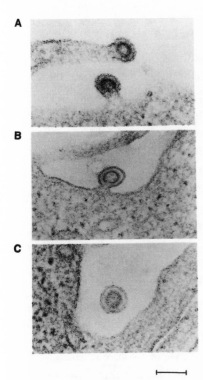

figure 11.1. *Porcine endogenous retrovirus particles budding from pig kidney cells. (The bar represents a distance of 100 nanometers. 1 nanometer = 0.000001 millimeter.) (Courtesy of Clive Patience, Ph.D. Reproduced with permission from* Nature Medicine 3, 275, 1997.)

hosts, or possibly combine with other human viruses or DNA, to produce a completely new pathogen with unpredictable biological properties that could include resistance to the human immune system. This possibility, however remote, is causing concern because, unlike the viruses that bring on a short-lived illness such as influenza, retroviral infection is lifelong but may remain quiescent for many years before causing cancer or an AIDS-like immuno-deficiency condition in the patient. Alternatively—or additionally—the pig virus might mutate or combine in the human host with a human virus, form-ing a new virus that is lethal to pigs rather than to humans. The release of this virus from a transplant recipient into the community might prove dis-astrous to the pig farming industry.

It is theoretically possible to breed an endogenous retrovirus out of a herd of pigs over many generations, or to "knock out" such genes by genetic techniques. However, these approaches will undoubtedly prove difficult, and if many retroviruses are found to be present, as seems likely, it may be im-possible. What is known to date—largely from the work of British virologists Robin Weiss and Clive Patience—is that the pig endogenous retroviruses that have been identified can, under certain ideal laboratory conditions, be transferred to human cells, which they then infect. Whether this can only take place in the laboratory or whether it will also occur if a pig organ is transplanted into a human remains unknown. It is also not known if pig endogenous retroviruses will cause any disease even if they do infect the cells of the human recipient. They may remain just as benign as in the pig. Current expert opinion is that this type of endogenous retrovirus is generally weak and does not fare well in a foreign environment, such as a host of another species. Even if they are successfully transferred to the human host's cells, it is believed unlikely that they would be transferred by contact to third parties. However, the potential for disease and illness in the form of cancer or possibly an AIDS-like condition is sufficient to warrant both caution and investigation before xenotransplantation moves ahead.

Investigations are under way to see if baboons and monkeys that receive pig organ transplants become infected by these pig retroviruses. At present, there is no evidence that this is occurring. This may indicate that the pig retrovirus will not infect human cells under the conditions associated with an organ transplant. Even if they do but remain healthy, this will be encouraging. However, a follow-up of several years may be needed to ascertain if the retroviruses are going to cause late problems. There are also a hundred or more patients scattered in various countries around the world who, at one time or another, have received a pig tissue graft—for example, pig islet and skin grafts. All of these grafts were in direct contact with the patients' body fluids and tissues for a period of time. Furthermore, the majority of these patients were receiving immunosuppressive drugs or were to some extent naturally immunosuppressed by the underlying disease process, for example, by the extensive burn that necessitated the pig skin graft. To date, none of these patients has been found conclusively to harbor a pig endogenous retrovirus.

The Human Factor o o o

The patients who receive pig organs or cells will require monitoring throughout their lifetimes. This is, of course, what occurs in any transplant patient today with a human organ. However, in view of the unknowns discussed above, the monitoring will be much more intensive in patients who receive a pig organ. Blood will be taken at intervals and stored for testing at a later date if a disease process develops. This need for lifelong monitoring forms the basis of the guidelines put forward by the U.S. Public Health Service and the U.K. Advisory Group on the Ethics of Xenotransplantation.

It has been suggested that, as a safeguard, a patient who receives an organ from a pig should be kept in isolation and observed for a period of

time to ensure that no infection has been transferred. However, the incubation period (the period of time from the introduction of the virus into the
body to the development of symptoms and signs of overt infection) of some
viruses may be many years, as is the case with HIV. It would clearly be im-
practical and inhumane, and probably illegal, to isolate the patient for this
length of time.

A compromise that has also been suggested would be to restrict the patient's contacts with others—perhaps to only hospital personnel and close
family—for a period of time. Protected sexual contact between patient and
partner would also be essential. But again, how long should such restrictions
last? It is impossible to answer this question with any accuracy.

Physicians will have to be on the alert not only for well-recognized features of infection but also for any abnormal symptoms in their transplant
patients that might indicate that an unusual infection is developing. Should
such abnormal signs develop, the patient will require investigation for all
known (and unknown) microbes, and the medical and nursing teams and all
close contacts of the patient (family and friends) will also require investigation for any signs of disease. Laboratory personnel who handled the animal
tissues before transplantation may also be at some risk for infection, although
this will be much more limited than for the patient. The risk will probably be
similar to that of commercial meat preparers and animal care or veterinary
personnel who are routinely exposed to pigs—unless a dangerous mutation
of the organism has occurred, in which case the risk might be far greater. To
follow up, or at least to keep in contact with, all of these people—patients,
family, friends, health care workers, animal handlers, and so on—will be an
immense, if not impossible, undertaking. When one considers the number
of contacts that the average person has over a number of years, including
close or intimate contacts, the scope of this task can be fully appreciated.

The Noncompliant Patient o o o

Even with firm guidelines and laws, it will prove difficult to keep track of the
health status of this myriad of people, particularly when such matters as
protection of their privacy and confidentiality have to be considered. The
family and friends of the patient, and even the patient him- or herself, may
at some stage refuse to be subjected to such monitoring. Compliance within
any patient group is far from 100%, and organ transplant recipients are no
exception. Every transplant center can identify patients who do not take their
drugs regularly, do not attend follow-up clinics, or do not report serious complications in a timely manner.

Human nature being what it is, it is inconceivable that all xenotransplantation patients and their contacts will adhere to the guidelines required of them no matter how well they are screened and prepared in the workup to the transplant. If recipients of pig organs are found to harbor hitherto unknown pig viruses that cause disease in humans, it may only take one noncompliant or irresponsible patient to begin the spread of that disease throughout the community, just as AIDS can be spread by similar individuals. There are therefore many ethical and legal questions that remain to be asked and resolved.

A Reason for Optimism o o o

It is ironic that although the potential infectious risks of xenotransplantation have been discussed intensely for the past several years at almost every medical and governmental level, xenotransplantation continues to take place in patients in the United States. For example, pig brain cells are currently being placed into the brains of patients with Parkinson's disease and epilepsy, and pig livers are being used for extracorporeal perfusion in patients with fulminant hepatic failure. Perhaps it seems odd that these trials are continuing while the risks outlined in this chapter continue to be discussed. These very trials, however, provide reason for optimism: to date, no infectious-disease transmission has been reported in these very carefully monitored patients. Indeed, in the light of the data and expert opinions collected by the Xenotransplantation Subcommittee set up by the U.S. Food and Drug Administration to review the topic, the personal opinion of the chairman of the subcommittee, Hugh Auchincloss Jr. was that "the likelihood of endangering the public health by xenotransplantation is remote."

chapter 12

Guinea Pigs

The selection of the first patients

Laboratory to Hospital:
When Do We Make the Leap? ○ ○ ○

Scientists are making gradual progress in overcoming the scientific hurdles that nature has set before them. But, as with most areas of medical advance, not all of the problems will be solved in one fell swoop. Initially we may be able to offer patients animal organs or cells that survive and function for periods of weeks or months. With time, experience, and new developments, this period will be extended to years and eventually decades.

This has been the case with the transplantation of human organs, the results of which have steadily improved over the years. Little more than 15 years ago, the one-year survival of patients who underwent heart transplantation was in the region of 50%, and the five-year survival only 20%. Today, 80 to 90% of patients survive at least 12 months, and the 10-year survival is approximately 50%.

When heart transplantation was first introduced in 1967 by Christiaan Barnard and his colleagues in Cape Town, the initial results obtained during the first few years were extremely poor by today's standards. Only 4 of his first 10 patients survived one year, although 2 survived over 10 years and one of these survived over 20 years, becoming, at over 23 years, the longest-surviving heart transplant patient to date. (One of us cared for this patient for more than seven years. Throughout this period he worked full time, came to the hospital for checkups only once every three months, and never required admission for problems related to his transplant.) It was, therefore, clearly worthwhile for these two long-term survivors to undergo the procedure, and probably also for the other two who survived more than one year, as their quality of life during that year was good. For the remainder, it is unlikely the operation contributed much either to the quantity or quality of their remaining days.

Almost certainly, the same situation will arise with regard to our initial efforts in xenotransplantation. A small percentage of the patients will benefit greatly, another small percentage will benefit moderately, but a majority may not benefit at all, except for the knowledge that they have paved the way for those who follow. They will be the guinea pigs for those in the future. Only through slowly learning the problems and the solutions will we be able to improve the management of the next generation of patients.

If there were no obvious problems that might bar this step forward, such as major concerns about possible transfer of infection to the patient and even to the public at large, at what stage should we embark on a clinical program of xenotransplantation? We cannot wait until we are assured of a one-year survival rate between 80 and 90% and a five-year survival rate of 50% because this will unfortunately not be achieved without the experience we gain through failure. If we do not attempt xenotransplantation in human patients, then we shall clearly never develop this experience.

Experimentation on animals will not provide us with all the answers we need. Human subjects frequently pose unique problems that are not met in any experimental model. For example, when the immunosuppressive agent cyclosporine was tested in animals, it was never found to have any toxic effects on the kidneys. In humans, however, it is quite strongly nephrotoxic, and in some of the early patients this led to rapid kidney failure and occasionally even to death. Dosages consequently had to be adjusted dramatically to avoid this problem. This could never have been sorted out in experimental animal models, as the problem never arose. Indeed, Sir Roy Calne, the first surgeon to investigate comprehensively the use of cyclosporine in the experimental animal and the first to use it in human patients, went so far as to say that if it had been shown to be as toxic in animals as it is in humans, the drug might never have gained regulatory approval. And yet, with modifications made to dosage when the problem became obvious, cyclosporine has proved to be perhaps the single most important factor in the good results being obtained by transplant programs today.

Human patients may also provide opportunities for progress that the experimental animal does not. It is frequently easier to manage a human patient, who can cooperate with his or her physicians, in a hospital setting, with all the facilities that this provides, than it is to manage a rat, dog, or baboon in a laboratory. The resources of even the best experimental laboratory never match those of a major hospital. The successful introduction of a new therapeutic modality may be easier to achieve in a hospital setting.

We must not think of delaying the move from the laboratory to the hospital until we have *all* of the problems solved. This happy state will never be achieved, no matter how much effort we exert, no matter how much preparation we make. Christiaan Barnard, who had learned this lesson, was emphatic in his advice. "You cannot stay in the laboratory forever," he would say. There comes a time when both the surgeon and the patient must have the courage to take that leap into the unknown. Without that leap, further progress will be impeded.

On the other hand, it would be quite unethical to make the leap from laboratory to hospital prematurely. Every reasonable effort must have been made in the laboratory to sort out the problems we face. It would be against all ethical principles to subject a patient to a new procedure that had been inadequately investigated in the laboratory. Furthermore, if our initial clinical efforts involve errors of judgment that could have been avoided by further experimental research, and which result in premature or poorly planned clinical trials or are accompanied by bad publicity related to failure of the science, then transplantation in general may fall into disrepute. One obvious backlash would be a reluctance of families of donors to donate cadaveric human organs.

One argument sometimes put forward by surgeons is that if they do not carry out a new procedure, such as xenotransplantation, their patient will die. Undoubtedly this is usually true. But it is surely unacceptable for surgeons and physicians to claim that they must proceed with an experimental clinical undertaking if that procedure is inadequately researched and developed. This might well result in the patient's suffering a drawn-out and painful death, rather than a relatively peaceful death with dignity.

Similarly, a surgeon cannot justify performing an inadequately researched or tested procedure on the grounds that the patient knows he or she is dying and is willing to take the risks involved. A dying patient is frequently desperate, and a desperate individual does not always make decisions in the best interests of society at large or even of patients as a group. Desperate people do not even always make decisions that are in their own best interests. Nevertheless, consideration must always be given to the patient who, accepting that death is near, knowingly and freely chooses to offer him- or herself as an experimental subject in the hope that this participation will be of value to medical science and will benefit others in the future.

Patients unfortunately die daily in large numbers from disorders for which we do not have a perfect (or even imperfect) therapy. Even with thorough investigation in the laboratory, xenotransplantation will certainly not be a perfect therapy for many years to come. We have to accept the fact that in the immediate future, our clinical efforts in this area will be of an experimental nature and cannot realistically be offered to the patient as a potential cure, likely to provide him or her with a good quality of life for a prolonged period of time. We hope and trust this step will come with time, but our initial efforts will surely be primarily to learn more of the science relating to this topic, and it is unfortunately unlikely that many of the early patients will benefit significantly.

Are We Ready for a Clinical Trial? ○ ○ ○

Medical ethicists Renee Fox and Judith Swazey have suggested that four criteria need to be fulfilled to justify any clinical trial: the need has to be established, an appropriate group of patients has to be identified, sufficient experimental advances must have taken place that justify the transfer of the technology from laboratory to hospital, and the ethical appropriateness of such a clinical trial has to be determined. Let us now consider the first three of these requirements. In the following chapter we shall discuss the last.

Undoubtedly, the clinical need for donor organs on a much larger scale than can be met by human cadaveric or living-related organ donation has been established, as we discussed in Chapter 2. Few would disagree with this conclusion.

Who Are the Most Likely Guinea Pigs? ○ ○ ○

Several groups of patients have been identified as being suitable as the initial subjects for animal organ transplants. They basically fall into two separate and distinct groups—those who have nothing to lose and those in whom it will do no harm. The first group is made up of dying patients for whom no alternative medical therapy is available. If the graft is not successful, the outcome to the patient will not have changed—he or she will unfortunately die. This group therefore seemingly has nothing to lose by the attempt. Conversely, the second group consists of patients who are not at immediate risk of dying and for whom some form of alternative medical therapy is available as a backup in the event of failure. Failure of the xenografted organ is not likely to result in their death. They will therefore likely survive whether or not they undergo the transplant.

As an example of the first group, a pig organ transplant could be offered to a patient with rapidly developing heart failure or fulminant liver failure. The animal organ could be transplanted to keep the patient alive until a suitable human organ became available, at which time it could be replaced. This would enable the medical team to gain experience with the short-term use of the xenograft without committing the patient to depend on the animal organ for months or years. As the patient will in all probability die without the graft, the patient could be judged to have lost nothing in the event that the organ fails. As experience is gained and lessons are learned, medical science would develop the skills and confidence to enable the xenografted organ to survive in the long term.

A patient in chronic kidney failure who is supported by regular dialysis would be an example of the second group. Failure of the xenograft would most likely not lead to death; the patient would return to regular dialysis and should therefore be no worse off for the experience. A suitable patient who would have much to gain if the xenograft were successful would be one in whom a human kidney transplant is precluded by a high degree of sensitization that would inevitably lead to rejection of a human kidney very rapidly.

Those who have nothing to lose

Robert Michler is a heart surgeon in Ohio who has had a long interest in xenotransplantation and has contributed significant research efforts in this field. He has put forward the case of infants and children requiring urgent heart transplantation. In contrast to adults, no mechanical cardiac assist devices (artificial hearts) are available to support these smallest patients. An animal heart would be utilized as a temporary "bridge" until a human heart became available. Many, however, would question whether experimental clinical procedures of this nature should initially be tested in infants and children, who are personally unable to give informed consent. Our own preference would be to perform the early clinical trials in adults. Indeed, this was also the conclusion of the U.K. Advisory Group on the Ethics of Xenotransplantation, which recommended that "children should not be included in trials, at least until all the initial concerns about safety and efficacy have been satisfactorily resolved."

If not children, who might these adult patients be? In an earlier chapter, we examined the predicament of the young patient in fulminant liver failure, from viral or other cause, who is rapidly deteriorating and who will suffer permanent brain injury if liver transplantation is delayed more than a few hours. The use of pig livers to provide extracorporeal support might prove the first step (as this avoids a major surgical procedure) in the effort to keep the patient alive until a human liver becomes available; indeed, this has been attempted in the past. Although a pig liver is unlikely to fulfill all of the functions required of it in a human, it may at least detoxify the body sufficiently to reverse the detrimental effects on the brain and allow the patient to survive for a few days longer. Several centers in the United Kingdom and United States are planning or beginning such programs of extracorporeal liver hemoperfusion, using pig livers transgenic for human complement-regulatory proteins, as a first step toward the goal of permanent organ xenotransplantation.

If extracorporeal liver perfusion proved successful, the experience gained might give us confidence to progress to the actual transplantation of a pig liver, possibly in an auxiliary position, as an interim bridge until a human cadaveric liver becomes available. This might be preferable to daily extracorporeal liver perfusions. When a human donor liver is available, the bridging pig liver would be removed.

Alternatively, an attractive candidate for our initial trial of xenotransplantation might be an adult urgently awaiting heart transplantation. A patient weighing over 200 lb (and particularly one with blood type O) may wait several *years* for a heart transplant as a donor heart of suitable size to support his or her circulation becomes available relatively rarely. If the patient is deteriorating significantly, the only options available would be the insertion of a mechanical cardiac assist device or possibly a cardiac xenotransplant. Either would initially be inserted as a temporary bridge until a human organ was found. The length of time the bridge would be expected to support the patient might, however, be prolonged, and may extend to several months or even a year or more.

A further group of patients who might prove candidates for this same approach would be hitherto healthy people—generally men—who suffer a sudden heart attack. A subgroup of these go into rapid heart failure over a few hours, and in this group there is an 80 to 90% mortality rate. These patients are not on the transplant waiting list, and even if they were, the chance of obtaining a human donor heart within the few hours of life that remain is negligible. Their only hope is an animal heart transplant or the insertion of a mechanical device.

As we have significantly more experience with mechanical assist devices than with the transplantation of animal hearts, it would be an ethically difficult decision to decide on a xenotransplant if a mechanical assist device were readily available. However, the disadvantages of an assist device are several. The patient's life is dependent on portable batteries or an electrical console. A wire connecting the implanted device with the external power source protrudes from the chest or abdomen, and always remains a risk for the entry of infection into the body. The metal and other surfaces of the mechanical device provide a continuing site for blood clots to form, with a risk, admittedly small, of a clot breaking away and being carried to the brain, resulting in a stroke. A transplanted animal heart will also carry significant risks of its own, not least being that of early rejection, but there may be circumstances, such as small size, in some patients that would favor a xeno-transplant rather than a mechanical device.

One option open to us would be to insert the pig organ as an auxiliary heart, leaving the patient's own heart in place. This would be intended to maintain life while the patient's own heart was given the opportunity to re-cover over a period of a few weeks. If it did, the pig heart could be removed. If not, the patient could undergo transplantation with a human heart when one became available, at which time the pig heart could be taken out. For example, we now have fairly considerable experience with the use of me chanical assist devices in patients who have just suffered a massive heart attack. We know that in a proportion of these patients, their hearts will even-tually recover, and the mechanical assist device can be removed.

This sounds like the ideal approach, and theoretically it might be, but from a practical perspective such plans do not always work out just as anticipated. For example, rejection of the auxiliary pig heart, or the in-creased immunosuppression necessary to treat it, might be associated with a complication that could jeopardize the patient's life. Kidney failure, for example, can occur if there is a degree of heart failure (from rejection) in a patient receiving high doses of certain immunosuppressive drugs, such as cyclosporine or tacrolimus. The onset of kidney failure in a patient who in any case is barely clinging to life might well tip the balance in the wrong direction. Nevertheless, it is an option to consider. And we also have to remember that, if one pig heart fails, there may be the option of implant-ing a second—there will always be an unlimited number of pig hearts available.

A further alternative would be to transplant the pig heart and use a me-chanical assist device if the pig heart is rejected. Ethically, however, it might be difficult to justify this approach; if a mechanical assist device is available and the patient is suitable for its use, why put the patient at the added risk of having a pig heart transplant first?

Any trial of such a bridging procedure would be embarked upon in the full knowledge that bridging in no way increases the number of potential human donors available, but only redistributes them. Furthermore, bridging generally necessitates only the sickest patients being subjected to the procedure, thus weighting the odds against success. Nevertheless, bridging would enable us to gain experience regarding the short-term function of the transplanted animal organ without preventing the patient from benefiting from a human organ transplant when one became available. One other important point: current evidence is that if the patient has been bridged by a pig organ for a few weeks and has developed new or high levels of anti-pig antibodies, this in no way precludes him or her from undergoing a subsequent transplant with a human organ.

In view of the shortage of suitable human organs, almost inevitably some bridged patients will have to be supported by the xenograft for a longer period of time than initially anticipated. Knowledge of the limits of function and survival of the transplanted animal organ will therefore steadily be gained, as will knowledge of the problems that will be faced. A further comparison in this respect with mechanical cardiac assist devices is apt. These devices, implanted as temporary support until a human heart could be transplanted, were initially required to function for only several days. With the increasing shortage of donor hearts, they were required for longer and longer periods of time, and in the occasional patient have acted as a bridge for a period in excess of a year. Based on this experience, some mechanical hearts are now being implanted with the intention that they will serve as permanent life support for the patient. In other words, the patient is not expecting an eventual heart transplant, but knows that his or her life depends on the good function of the mechanical device. The transplantation of pig hearts may well follow a similar evolution.

There are cardiologists and cardiac transplant surgeons, however, who believe that xenotransplantation should be offered as a permanent form of therapy to patients in heart failure who, for one reason or another, are not considered suitable candidates for human heart transplantation. These might include some elderly patients, those with severe and widespread atherosclerotic disease, those with advanced diabetes, and others who have been turned down for a place on the transplant list. If supportive drug therapy is not maintaining them, they might have no other option but to take the risk of a xenograft. If a transplanted pig heart could keep them alive only for a year or so, but the quality of life during this period was good, many would consider this an option worth choosing.

In Chapter 2 we highlighted the plight of a patient with a transplanted human donor organ that was failing from chronic rejection. Remember that this happens within about 10 years to approximately 50% of those with an organ transplant. Many of these patients will have developed complications from long-term immunosuppressive drug therapy, such as weak bones, mild to moderate diabetes, or some degree of kidney failure. Or they might have suffered from progression of their underlying disease. For example, the patient with widespread atherosclerosis—hardening of the arteries—might have undergone a heart transplant because of coronary artery disease, but since then he might have also suffered blockage of the artery to the leg or a stroke from blockage of an artery to part of the brain. Although he may remain active and be enjoying life, he may no longer be an ideal candidate for a second transplant. His surgeon may not feel able to justify the use of a second scarce resource, a human donor heart, in a patient who is less likely to do as well the second time around. Such patients, however, might jump at the chance of a pig heart transplant. At least this would give them a second opportunity—and it would do so without depriving a first-time candidate of the chance to receive a human donor heart. Indeed, in order to distribute human organs fairly, a case could be made for limiting *all* retransplants to the use of pig organs—at least until such time as the results of pig organ transplants are equivalent to those of human organs.

Those in whom it will do no harm

Chapter 5 discussed the development of antibodies against human tissues in some patients with long-standing kidney disease. It may take many years to find such a patient a human donor kidney which will not be hyperacutely rejected. The presence of the antibodies, which result from previous pregnancy, blood transfusion, or kidney transplant, causes rapid destruction of the newly transplanted human kidney. The mechanism of graft destruction is virtually identical to that which happens when a pig organ is transplanted into an unmodified human recipient, but the two sets of antibodies—anti-human allograft (anti-HLA) and anti-pig xenograft (anti-Gal)—are quite different. Present evidence suggests that the fact that the patient has developed anti-human antibodies in no way complicates his or her having a pig organ xenograft. A pig kidney transplant may therefore be the only hope such a patient will ever have of getting off the treadmill of requiring dialysis with the artificial kidney machine three or four times a week, year in and year out. These patients should therefore be high on the list of potential candidates for a pig kidney transplant. Indeed, such highly sensitized patients, as well as patients who for technical reasons cannot continue with regular dialysis support, may have no alternative but pig kidney transplantation. Current opinion among surgeons and physicians interested in xenotransplantation is that this group of patients will indeed be the very first to be offered the opportunity of permanent pig organ xeno-transplantation.

But what if we attempt to get our initial experience not in patients requiring a whole-organ transplant but in those requiring only the transplantation of specialized cells or tissues? The risks for these patient are far smaller than for those requiring the transplant of a life-supporting organ, though the rewards of success may also be less dramatic.

The relatively rare "brittle" diabetic patients who cannot be managed satisfactorily medically by frequent insulin injections but whose diabetes might be controlled by the implantation of pig pancreatic islet cells form one group that would undoubtedly benefit from successful xenotransplantation. They could then throw away their insulin syringes and lead much more normal lives, the pig islet cells producing insulin when their bodies need it. Those of us who are fortunate enough not to need to inject ourselves once, twice, or maybe more times each and every day of our lives cannot appreciate, or even contemplate, what a relief it must be to be free of such uncomfortable injections once and for all. It must be like the released prisoner who is able to throw off his shackles and start life anew.

Trials of pig islets in such human patients have already been carried out by surgeons in Sweden and in New Zealand. So the modern era is already upon us, as these trials have been followed by others (Table 12.1), involving, for example, the injection of cow chromaffin cells into the spinal cord in the

table 12.1

Current or Recent Clinical Trials in Xenotransplantation in the United States and Europe

Patient's Disease	Tissues/Cells Transplanted	Donor Species
Liver failure	1. Hepatocytes*	Pig
	2. Whole liver*	Pig
Diabetes mellitus	Pancreatic islets	Pig
Degenerative neurological diseases	1. Neuronal cells	Pig
	2. Engineered kidney cells	Hamster
AIDS (HIV-1)	Bone marrow cells	Baboon
Refractory pain (terminal cancer)	Adrenal (chromaffin) cells	Cow

*Patient's blood perfused ex vivo through an artificial liver (consisting of isolated pig cells) or through a whole pig liver (which is not actually transplanted into the patient's body).

treatment of patients with intractable pain and the injection of specialized pig brain cells into the human brain in the hope of reversing the symptoms of neurodegenerative diseases.

There are therefore several clearly identified groups of appropriate patients who might be considered for our first attempts at the transplantation of animal organs or tissues. In the case of tissue or cell transplants, these patients are already being selected and undergoing xenotransplantation. In the case of whole-organ transplants, we yet have to make these difficult decisions.

Assessing the patient

Whichever patients are selected to participate in the early clinical trials, it will be essential to first subject them to a careful psychosocial assessment. The intention would be not only to ensure that they are freely and genuinely motivated to participate and are not being subjected to undue pressure from members of the surgical team, family, or others interested in their well-being, but also to ensure that if the transplant is a success, they could cope with their newfound situation.

Will the existence of a pig organ in their body affect their self-image or cause unexpected stress? Will they feel that their dignity is diminished by having an animal organ? As the report of the Nuffield Council on Bioethics in the United Kingdom pointed out, "It is difficult to predict how people's views of their bodies and of their identities might be affected by xenotransplantation. On the one hand, the use of animal organs might eliminate any disturbing implications associated with receiving a human organ. On the other hand, receiving an animal transplant might cause different stresses. The response is likely to reflect emotions of what it is to be a person, to be human, and to be an animal. These notions are not uniform for this or any other society, but vary according to social and cultural background."

In other words, some patients with a pig heart functioning within their chest could look their spouse/lover in the eye and, perhaps with a grin, say, "I love you with all my heart." Possibly a few, however, would choke on the words and find the very thought deeply embarrassing and psychologically disturbing.

It could be pointed out that pig heart valves have been implanted in patients for more than 20 years and, by and large, have given rise to few serious psychological problems. But pig valves are small pieces of tissue that have been treated to make them nonviable. That someone might respond psychologically more strongly to the transplant of a vital organ, such as the heart, is more likely. Certainly occasional patients suffer considerable psychological trauma from the fact that they have another person's organ in their body, although this is usually related to feelings of guilt that they have benefited from another's unfortunate death.

Is the Technology Ready? ○ ○ ○

What results do we need to see in the experimental laboratory in order to warrant moving on to treat patients? In other words, has the technology been sufficiently proven in the laboratory for us to believe it might be successful when applied to a human patient? Although much experimental work in transplantation biology is carried out in laboratory rats or mice, work in rodents is insufficient as a basis for human clinical trials. It is usually essential to obtain significant experience in the much more closely related and relevant nonhuman primate experimental model. This is particularly so if we plan to use the pig as the donor, in view of the very important immunological differences between higher primates (including humans), on the one hand, and lower mammals (including the pig), on the other.

If the intention is to utilize the animal organ only as a temporary bridge to support life until a human organ becomes available, the results we should be seeing in the laboratory need perhaps be only relatively modest. To proceed to the use of extracorporeal liver perfusion in patients dying of fulminant hepatic failure, all we need to demonstrate is that a pig liver will provide a detoxifying function for the patient over the course of a few hours. We also need to have demonstrated that repeated liver perfusions, continued over several days, would be tolerated and not be detrimental to the patient. That has in fact been demonstrated several times in the past.

If we are planning to use a pig heart as a bridge for a human heart, then we should at least be able to demonstrate *consistently* satisfactory function of the xenografted organ in an experimental model (for example, of a pig heart in a baboon) for a minimum period of, say, four weeks. In the clinical setting, this might well provide sufficient time for a human organ to be obtained to replace the temporary pig organ. Furthermore, the experimental model used would require that the recipient animal be totally supported by the donor organ. To demonstrate, for example, function of an auxiliary pig heart in a baboon, where the pig heart does not support the baboon's circulation, would be insufficient evidence that a heart transplanted in the normal position in the chest would support the life of a patient for the same period of time. We would need to have carried out a series of experiments where the baboon's heart was removed and replaced by the pig heart. If a series of 10 or so consecutive baboons survived this procedure for a month or more without developing major complications from the therapy required, then we could be optimistic that a group of patients might survive also.

If the organ is planned to be used as a permanent replacement, then we need to demonstrate repeatedly and consistently in the laboratory that the transplanted organ will support life for a minimum period of, say, six months or a year, and preferably longer. Even periods of a year or more may be an insufficient test. But the difficulties associated with maintaining an uncommunicative animal with a life-supporting organ transplant are considerable when compared with supporting a similar human patient, as we discussed earlier in this chapter. Six months' follow-up would provide sufficient information to expect at least comparable success in the patient. One must remember that it is not just the length of survival of the organ that we are interested in. Biopsies of the organ can be taken at intervals, and if there are no features of rejection throughout the entire period of follow-up, we could feel encouraged that whatever therapy was being provided was successful. Many blood tests could also be performed, the results of which would also indicate the extent of the success of the therapy. If, on the other hand, the biopsies and blood tests demonstrated repeated rejection episodes that required extra therapy throughout the six-month period, then, even if the organ survived, the wisdom of progressing to the treatment of patients would need to be reconsidered. In this event, a longer period of observation in the laboratory may be required to document survival at one or two years before a final decision could be made regarding a clinical trial.

In contrast, a period of observation shorter than six months might prove acceptable under certain circumstances. For example, if immunological tolerance had clearly been achieved in the recipient animal and therefore no immunosuppressive therapy was required, the quality of life of the animal was excellent with no episodes of infection, and repeated biopsies of the transplanted organ demonstrated no signs of rejection, then a follow-up period as short as three months might be deemed sufficient to warrant testing this therapy in humans. In any event, the experience in the animal model would need to be sufficient to allow us insight into the functioning of the donor organ in its unusual environment. Potential physiological incompatibilities, particularly of the xenotransplanted kidney or liver, may be revealed during this period.

The final question is what results would we expect and require from the initial few xenotransplants in human patients to warrant continuing such transplants in a larger group of patients. If bridging was successful and kept the patient alive until a human organ could be transplanted, then further bridging procedures could be planned. Alternatively, if animal organs are initially placed as intended permanent grafts, and if a significant percentage of the first small group of patients survive for more than one year with an acceptable quality of life (and without proving to be an infection hazard to others), then this would encourage us to continue with the procedure as a therapeutic option for other carefully selected patients.

When Will It Happen? ○ ○ ○

At the present time, a clinical trial using a baboon as the donor might well be relatively successful, with such organs surviving for several months or longer in human recipients. Even if successful, however, the use of baboon organs will never resolve the fundamental problem of the inadequacy of the number of donor organs available for transplantation. It can at best be an interim measure (from which we would undoubtedly gain valuable knowledge) until we solve the problems relating to the use of the pig as a donor. If it will prove only an interim measure, and in view of the potential risks of infection associated with the transplantation of nonhuman primate organs into humans, such a clinical trial of baboon organ transplants is unjustified. It remains possible, however, that, in the absence of a global prohibition of such a procedure, one or more surgeons somewhere may be tempted to embark upon such a trial during the next few years. It would be wiser, however, to await further laboratory progress in the transplantation of pig organs.

Our prediction is that the first step will be the use of livers from pigs transgenic for a human complement regulatory protein, such as DAF, as extracorporeal life support; one such trial has already been initiated. The transplantation of permanent pig organs, such as the kidney, will probably not begin until the results of the liver support trials have been fully assessed, which may take a year or two. Furthermore, this period will be required to improve the science relating to the protection of the transplanted organ from the various rejection insults that the human body can inflict on it. Questions relating to the safety of xenotransplantation from a microbiological perspective also require clarification. Neither of these problems has yet been resolved, and resolution is necessary before a clinical trial could be justified. But knowledge in both fields is progressing rapidly, and the liver support trials will provide further important data.

The above predictions, however, may prove to be perfect examples of those that are "risky, especially about the future," and we are resigned to being proven wrong, one way or the other.

chapter 13

Animal Rights and Human Wrongs

Ethical concerns

The Ethics of a Clinical Trial ○ ○ ○

Although we might agree on which patients should be offered xenotransplantation first, let us consider further whether we are ready to embark on this next giant leap for mankind. The ethical appropriateness of initiating such clinical trials is intricately intertwined with many factors, not least the state of the science. Indeed, if the science is sufficiently advanced and the potential benefit to patients seems assured, then it may be unethical and irresponsible *not* to initiate clinical trials. In contrast, if the science is insufficiently advanced and patients are unlikely to benefit therapeutically from the procedure, then the trial is inappropriate.

Let us examine the status of xenotransplantation science. Only a few organs transplanted between closely related animals—such as a monkey kidney or heart transplanted into a baboon—have functioned for more than a few months. We therefore have virtually no data on what might happen to such grafts in the long term. Unless a technique for inducing immunological tolerance can be perfected, such xenografts would require a heavy and prolonged regimen of immunosuppression. These drugs would significantly increase the risk of major, possibly fatal, infectious complications as well as increase the incidence of certain types of cancer. The early development of chronic rejection remains likely. Baboon-to-human organ transplantation would also present other risks, such as the potential for the spread of a serious viral infection from the donor not only to the patient but also to his or her contacts. The use of primate organs would in any case be an interim measure until we perfect pig-to-human transplantation.

With regard to human trials of pig organs, current experimental results are too poor to justify trials at this time. (The only exceptions are cell transplants and the use of extracorporeal pig liver perfusion to bridge patients dying of fulminant hepatic failure.) Although we are likely to obtain function of a pig organ in a human for a few days or weeks, the pool of experimental data is presently insufficient to support the concept of *consistent* prolonged organ function. Because the risks associated with cell and tissue xenotransplantation are greatly reduced compared to those of the whole organ, trials in patients should be pursued, and in fact, a number of studies involving the transplantation of animal cells are already under way in the United States and Europe (see Table 12.1).

As the science gradually advances—which it is steadily doing—other factors will come into play. There are potential risks relating to most medical advances, some of which can be identified before the first patients are treated, and others that may become apparent only after clinical trials are already in progress.

The potential risk that has gained most attention in recent months is the possibility of introducing serious infection—a xenozoonosis—not only into the patient but into the general population. This topic has been fully discussed in Chapter 11; suffice it to say here that if transplant immunology progresses to the point where pigs can realistically solve the shortage of donor organs, then it would seem reasonable and ethical to transplant such organs—at least in a small initial group of patients—as long as the presence of all *known* microorganisms that could pose a threat to humans has been excluded. Adequate follow-up to detect hitherto unknown ones will also be required.

Animal Rights o o o

Is it ethical to use animals as sources of replacement parts for humans? A discussion of this topic could take up an entire volume. The human race has not always had the same concern for animals that it has today. It was only in the 19th century that attention began to be paid to the way animals were housed and treated. Legislation regarding animals was part of the social reform movement associated with such other matters as the abolition of slavery, the regulation of child and adult labor, improvement of prison conditions, and reform of education.

The use of animals for medical research is a topic on which many hold strong views. (It is perhaps ironic that so much time is spent debating this issue when so little is devoted to serious consideration of the estimated 10 to 16 million unwanted pets that are euthanized in the United States annually.) However, xenotransplantation does not raise the same ethical questions as the use of animals for medical research. These animals would not be subjected to experimentation, but would live in excellent conditions until humanely euthanized in the effort to save a person's life. Nevertheless, the prospect of xenotransplantation will almost certainly mobilize extremists from various animal groups. U.S. heart transplant surgeon Leonard Bailey was advised to wear a bulletproof vest after he received death threats following his involvement in the Baby Fae operation in 1984. The strength of feeling about the use of animals for medical purposes is illustrated by the fact that the hospital where Baby Fae was treated received 13,000 letters from the public protesting the use of a baboon as a donor, and yet only 75 were concerned with perceived misuse of the baby.

The attitude of at least some animal rights activists is illustrated by the experience of the surgical team at the University of Pittsburgh that performed two baboon liver transplants in patients in 1992 and 1993. Surgeon Tom Starzl, the leader of the team, had his home picketed and was branded as "Dr. Frankenstarzl," despite the fact that his massive contributions to the development of both human kidney and liver transplantation have saved countless lives. It must also be remembered that saving human lives was the aim of the baboon liver transplants.

Those who breed animals for organ donation will be regulated by various government bodies to ensure that the animals receive proper care and housing. The high quality of the end product—the donor organs—will be essential if such breeders are to remain in business. Since the livelihood of the breeders will depend on their raising healthy animals, the animals will be raised under ideal conditions that will certainly exceed those of all farm animals (and even some humans). Indeed, it is unlikely that any animals will ever have been maintained so carefully, with the possible exception of valuable racehorses.

When the time comes for organ retrieval, this will be carried out humanely under full anesthesia. The animal will die while anesthetized. Slaughterhouse animals will be expressly banned from use for organ or tissue donation, at least in the United States and most other Western countries, for fear of potential infectious contamination. There will therefore be important differences between animals bred for organ donation and those bred (or captured from the wild) for food consumption or medical or pharmaceutical research. For example, even if research animals are treated as humanely as possible, they may undergo surgical and other invasive and stressful procedures and perhaps receive drugs with potential side effects and complications. As a result, the arguments against the use of animals as donors of organs for humans should be significantly fewer than those directed against the use of animals in medical research.

Perhaps surprisingly, therefore, the U.K. Advisory Group on the Ethics of Xenotransplantation concluded that "it would be ethically unacceptable to use primates as source animals for xenotransplantation, not least because they would be exposed to too much suffering." Yet, in contrast, the advisory group deemed it "ethically acceptable to use primates in the research into xenotransplantation"—although they did add a rider stating that the animals should be used in research only "where no alternative method of obtaining information exists and this use should be limited as far as is possible."

Human attitudes toward animals have changed greatly through the centuries, and still vary between cultures. Even within a given society, opinions extend from one extreme, that humans can treat animals as they wish, to the other, that animals have rights equal to humans'. The middle-of-the-road view held by the majority is that animals should be treated humanely and with respect but are not entitled to the same rights as humans. Most of us would also accept that the more distant the species is from us phylogenetically (or in evolutionary terms), the fewer rights it has. (A notable exception is provided by endangered species; when threatened by extinction, their rights increase substantially.) The laboratory mouse, for example, would not have the same rights as a chimpanzee, but in contrast, would have more rights than an earthworm. By "rights" most of us mean that the animal is entitled to be treated as we would treat our fellow human. We provide better food, make greater efforts to prevent boredom and discomfort, and have more social contact with a pet dog (in whom we see many human traits) than with, for example, a mouse or an earthworm. In fact, we treat an animal more like a human—that is, we assign it greater value—to the extent that we believe it resembles us or displays human traits. James Walters, a contemporary philosopher, believes we can put animals on what can be loosely described as a "personhood scale," and thus grant highest moral status to those animals which we think are most like us.

This concept does not necessarily infer that a member of one animal species is always inferior to a member of another, even if the comparison is being made with humans. For example, a healthy chimpanzee may be an important interactive member of a social group or extended family of chimpanzees; since it demonstrates a degree of intelligence and emotion with which we can identify, it may be a "worthier" member of the animal world than, for example, a severely brain-damaged patient who has been in a vegetative state for many years, or an anencephalic infant, born without a major part of the brain.

If chimpanzees were available in large enough numbers to serve as donors for the transplant community, then our ethical quandary would be greatly increased. Many members of society, ourselves included, would have very severe reservations about killing chimpanzees or other great apes to act as donors of organs for humans. This would be particularly questionable in view of the fact that most countries do not allow the use of human anencephalic infants as organ donors.

Indeed, Christiaan Barnard, after inserting a chimpanzee heart into a patient, planned further transplants using chimpanzee donors. He quickly abandoned the idea, however, as, in his own words, "I became too attached to the chimpanzees." Abdul Daar, transplant surgeon and ethicist, has pointed out that if subhuman primates are genetically so close to us, then "they must have some of our rights, one of the most basic of which is not to be killed." (With lower species such as pigs, however, Daar suggests we should be more concerned with "animal welfare" rather than "animal rights.")

Our concerns are perhaps slightly lessened when we move down the evolutionary scale to animals such as the baboon, which are a little further removed from the human race. Nevertheless, the baboon has many human-like behavioral qualities, and the use of large numbers of such animals for xenotransplantation would certainly be unacceptable to many. Perhaps fortunately for society (and the baboon), current opinion is that they are unsuitable as organ donors for humans, as outlined in Chapter 4.

Our ethical qualms relating to the use of the pig as a donor animal are very much reduced in view of the fact that the pig is already purpose-bred as a source of food. Indeed, it has been suggested that the use of a pig as an organ donor—rather than as a mere provider of meat—is a "nobler" use of the animal. Furthermore, we have utilized pig insulin, pig heart valves and even pig skin in humans for many years. With regard to animal rights, the "bottom line" as far as the pig is concerned is that in order to provide us with food, insulin, or heart valves, the pig has to be killed. Those who do not object to slaughtering pigs for these purposes should surely have no objection to using the pig's organs or tissues for transplantation. And if we can employ pig heart valves in large numbers, then surely we should be able to make use of the animal's entire heart. We would suggest that only the strictest vegetarians, who do not eat any form of animal tissue, do not wear leather shoes, and so on, can reasonably raise objections to the use of the pig in xenotransplantation.

The "Humanized" Pig o o o

The use of transgenic or otherwise genetically engineered pigs, however, raises additional concerns. There are those who believe that genetic engineering is little different from selective breeding and should be considered as such. Pigs can be selected for a particular physical or biological trait, such as skin color or tender meat. By breeding from pigs that express that trait, all the pigs in the herd will have the trait within a few generations. The selected trait could, of course, be related to the needs of xenotransplantation. Genetic engineering allows us to achieve this goal much more rapidly. But it also allows us to breed genetically manipulated pigs that would be impossible to obtain by selective breeding. Pigs with human complement-regulatory proteins are one such example. In turn, cloning may prove a more efficient way of generating a herd of genetically modified animals. It therefore seems rather simplistic to compare genetic engineering with selective breeding.

We are already engineering pigs that express, at the least, a small amount of human protein (for example, a human complement-regulatory protein) or sugar in their organs. For all intents and purposes, this type of pig, albeit transgenic, remains very much a pig. But under what circumstances is a genetically altered pig no longer solely a pig? Some might consider this an intriguing philosophical question worthy of much debate; others may believe it too ridiculous even to ask. Regardless of the prevailing viewpoint, at some time in the future it is likely that ethical and even legal questions will be raised with regard to this matter.

Patrick Dixon, author of *The Genetic Revolution,* has pointed out that, as humans and monkeys differ by only approximately 2% in their genes, a transfer of just 0.5% could be highly significant. "We now have the technology to produce a 50:50 mix of any mammals we like. . . . How many human genes does an animal have to have to gain human rights?" Undoubtedly there will be those who will claim that such transgenic pigs have at least some human rights.

The U.K. Advisory Group on the Ethics of Xenotransplantation concluded that "some degree of genetic modification is ethically acceptable" but that "there are limits to the extent to which an animal should be genetically modified." It did not indicate what those limits might be. This was possibly sensible, as the limits are extremely difficult to define. For example, in a later valiant effort to do so, Ian Kennedy, the chairman of the group, suggested that pigs should not be "genetically manipulated beyond a point that we would regard as intolerable to the animal (a moral point of view, concerned with the *pigness* of pigs, which comes a point where the pig is no longer a pig and which might be deemed to be offensive to all)." We perhaps know vaguely what he means, but in practical scientific terms, what he says gives us no real guidance.

In the Netherlands, a committee has been set up to oversee all work involving biotechnology and animals. Acceptability of any proposed experiment involving animals is based on two guidelines. First, there must be no unacceptable implications for the health and welfare of the animal. Second, there must be no serious ethical objections to the procedure. This would presumably rule out alterations to the brain that might modify the thinking capacity of the pig (or of a human recipient of pig cells) or genetic changes that might lead to the reproduction of one species by the other. Any hint of the creation of the hideous chimeric creatures envisioned in H. G. Wells' novel *The Island of Doctor Moreau* must clearly be avoided.

The cloning of animals such as the pig raises many of the same ethical questions as does genetic engineering. The cloning of *humans*, however, raises an entirely new array of ethical dilemmas. This topic was given a sense of immediacy in late 1998 by a report that a human cell nucleus had been transferred into a cow ovum. A full discussion of this topic is clearly beyond the scope of this book. Suffice it to say that the potential ability to clone an individual human, or even a greatly modified human with less mental capacity than is normal, to provide organs for transplantation has spurred many to call for a ban on human cloning. In the United States, California has already banned human cloning, and similar legislation has been introduced in 24 other states. Furthermore, at least 19 nations have already signed an anti-cloning treaty. However, the potential of human cell cloning for research purposes and possibly to provide infertile couples with a much-wanted child or a child in whom a harmful gene has been deleted are seen by some as powerful arguments against such a blanket ban. Each new advance in biotechnology will bring further dilemmas that require answers.

The Public Attitude ○ ○ ○

The public's attitude toward any medical advance is clearly important. However, as with any aspect of our society (for example, abortion, pornography, capital punishment, and so on), attitudes may change over a period of time. Furthermore, the way of thinking tends to differ from one country to another or even within different regions of the same country. For example, as we mentioned earlier, the donation of organs from brain-dead individuals is not yet fully accepted in Japan, unlike in Western nations. The prevailing attitude within a community therefore needs to be carefully appraised. A potential medical or scientific "advance," even if likely to be successful, may be unacceptable to a particular community. To proceed with (or promote) such a step would undoubtedly be counterproductive under such adverse circumstances.

Our preconceptions about certain groups are not always confirmed by inquiry. Although both Moslem and Judaic laws prohibit the eating of pork (unless life depends on it), neither religion would appear to prohibit the transplantation of pig organs. (Perhaps this highly practical attitude toward pigs reflects to some extent the human attitude to many aspects of life. Our attitude about even strictly held principles changes when our backs are against the wall. The occasional reports of cannibalism by those stranded in remote places is one such example.) The fundamental teachings of other religious groups, such as Buddhists and Jains, make them opposed to xenotransplantation mainly on the grounds of their responsibility to protect animals, or at least not to injure them.

What is the public's attitude toward xenotransplantation in North America and Europe? In 1993 the Partnership for Organ Donation published a Gallup poll on the American public's attitude toward organ donation and transplantation. Of 6,127 people surveyed, 85% expressed general support for organ donation, and 79% stated that they would personally accept a human organ if they needed one. Furthermore, 50% approved the principle of xenotransplantation and stated they would accept an animal organ if a suitable human donor were not available.

It should be remembered, however, that these were the opinions of healthy men and women. They were not infirm, and presumably did not really think they would ever need an organ transplant. Our own opinion, based on many years caring for patients, is that if the survey had been carried out among patients awaiting organ transplantation, particularly those who were in an intensive care unit and staring death in the face, the percentage that would be prepared to accept an animal organ would have been much higher. On the basis of this survey, therefore, it would appear that there is already considerable support for xenotransplantation among the public.

The U.S. National Kidney Foundation and the newsletter *Transplant News* surveyed 7,900 transplant recipients, patients, families, and health care professionals. Of approximately 2,000 responses received, 1,400 were recipients of kidney transplants and 500 were nonrecipients. Almost 90% of both groups were aware of xenotransplantation research, and 65% agreed with such research. Seventy-four percent of the kidney recipients said they would have accepted a xenograft if no human organ had been available; interestingly, 85% said that the species of the donor animal would not have affected their decision. A survey of patients in the United Kingdom, carried out by David Poulter—a patient himself—provided a similar result, with 75% of patients polled "strongly supporting the research and its concepts." In a small survey of 238 high school students in the United Kingdom, 55% thought that research to develop pig organs for transplantation should continue.

Recent reports from the Institute of Medicine of the U.S. National Academy of Sciences and from the Institute of Biology and the Nuffield Council on Bioethics, both in the United Kingdom, seem to reflect the public attitude. They have been positive in accepting the idea that, to meet the growing demand for donor organs, xenotransplantation is ethical. The Institute of Medicine explored the attitudes toward xenotransplantation of individuals who were under the stress of awaiting a donor organ. The results are exemplified by the mother of a young man in urgent need of a liver transplant. The surgical team caring for her son raised the possibility of using a pig liver for extracorporeal perfusion as a temporary life-saving support. As the young man was too ill to make the decision himself, it fell to his mother. Her response was, "When they offered me the pig, I didn't think about the fact that it was a pig. I thought, 'We are losing this battle, and desperate men take desperate measures.' We were desperate. . . . I was going to do everything I possibly could to see him through this."

Not all surveys have been so positive. In a survey of 15,000 people in Europe, only 36% thought xenotransplantation was morally acceptable. In France, 48% of members of the public polled by telephone were against xenotransplantation. In Australia, where research into xenotransplantation is particularly active, no fewer than 66% of acute-care nurses were opposed to it. In a separate poll, less than 50% of renal dialysis or transplant patients were strongly in favor of xenotransplantation. A small U.K. study of potential renal transplant recipients indicated that 40% would accept a pig kidney, which presumably means that 60% were either undecided or would not accept the organ. Perhaps, however, patients with kidney disease do not reflect those truly in a life-or-death situation. Thrice-weekly support by an artificial kidney nearly always sustains life for a little longer. Such a luxury is not available to the patient awaiting a heart, liver, or lung transplant.

We are reminded of a former patient of one of us who was advised he needed a heart transplant rather urgently. Much earlier in life he had decided that he would never donate his organs or those of any member of his family. He therefore felt it morally wrong to accept an organ from a stranger, and decided against heart transplantation. After being resuscitated from his second cardiac arrest, however, he changed his mind. Strongly held views can rapidly become overturned when the grim reaper knocks on one's door. The patient, who became a close friend, underwent a successful heart transplant and, to his credit, has spent much of the past 10 years in making others aware of the urgent need for donor organs.

This change of heart—excuse the pun—is further demonstrated by the results of a poll of 1,200 people carried out by the Southeastern Institute of Research, a market research company based in Richmond, Virginia. Almost two-thirds of those polled believed that xenotransplantation research should continue. Of those "strongly opposed," however, no less than one-quarter said they would still consider a xenograft if no alternative were available.

An interesting observation made by the Gallup organization was raised by the Institute of Medicine committee. The committee drew attention to the disparities in the attitudes of those surveyed. Although 85% expressed support for human organ donation, only 52% of the respondents had actually made a personal decision to donate organs, and only 28% had ever formally given permission for organ donation. The committee suggested that this discrepancy was the result of fears and suspicions relating to the use of human organs. Although it remains uncertain whether the use of animal organs will be associated with similar fears and suspicions, successful xenotransplantation will eliminate the perceived problems relating to the use of human organs. These are, in fact, numerous.

For example, the concept of brain death is still poorly understood by many members of the public, a significant percentage of whom still have reservations and doubts about it. At intervals, reports emanate from such places as the Middle East, India, and South and Central America of entrepreneurial trafficking in human organs, in which living donors appear to have been exploited. Wild rumors crop up from time to time, particularly from Latin America, of homeless young people being murdered for their organs. Concerns have also been raised about practices in China, where most transplanted organs come from executed prisoners.

Amnesty International estimates that approximately 6,000 prisoners are executed in China each year. Chinese law allows the harvesting of their organs for humane medical purposes only if the donations are voluntary. However, human rights activists claim that authorities rarely ask the prisoners or their family for permission beforehand. According to *Time* magazine (March 9, 1998), they simply take whatever organs or tissue are needed after an execution. "Doctors at military hospitals then reportedly transplant the organs into wealthy foreigners." Particular concern has been expressed over the possible harvesting of organs from political prisoners, and that the kinds of crimes punishable by death may have increased in order to line the pockets of Chinese officials. In fact, FBI agents recently arrested two Chinese nationals for allegedly trying to sell organs of executed Chinese prisoners for hard currency. During the sting operation, the former Chinese prosecutor and his accomplice were secretly videotaped haggling over the price of various organs—the going rate seems to be around $20,000 for a kidney and $40,000 for a liver.

If kidneys, livers, or lungs are needed, the prisoner is shot through the back of the head, after which the "donor" is rushed to a mobile operating room and the organs are removed; if corneas are needed, the prisoner is shot in the chest. According to the Transplantation Society, the leading international medical society in this field, on one occasion, when the heart continued to beat, after some delay the prisoner was re-executed. An account was also received of a prisoner from whom *both* kidneys were removed in an operation the day *before* he was executed.

Although it is illegal to buy or sell human organs in the United States and many other countries, some individuals feel there is nothing ethically wrong in using organs from prisoners who are going to die anyway. The Transplantation Society, however, has taken a strong stand against this practice, and has threatened to cancel the membership of anyone found to have assisted Chinese transplant surgeons in this respect in any way. To add to the controversy, a new "life-for-a-life" bill has been introduced in the Missouri state legislature. This bill would allow death-row prisoners to donate an organ in exchange for a sentence of life imprisonment without parole. Although the prisoners would not technically be selling their organs, some ethicists argue that a choice between death and organ donation represents a form of coercion rather than a free choice.

Whether the families who donate organs from their brain-dead relatives should be compensated financially has been discussed for many years in Western countries but has remained a controversial issue. It has been suggested that the organ procurement organizations (OPOs) or the state should provide the organ donor's family with a "death benefit" of, say, a few hundred dollars, and Pennsylvania is in fact pursuing this approach. In our materialistic Western society, this reward might well act as an incentive to families to consider donation more carefully. It seems to work in Spain, which has the highest organ donation rate in the world, where the funeral expenses of the donor can be legally paid by the OPO. (Other financial factors, however, may also play important roles as the Spanish government offers incentives to both the donor hospital and to specified physicians who identify potential donors and obtain family consent for donation.) But cogent arguments against what some see as "twisting their arms" in this way have been put forward. The view of some critics is that money corrupts, and many see this as a way of influencing the poor but not the wealthy. However, there are others who believe that such a system should be given a fair trial. Our own guess is that, whatever its faults, the prospect of financial reward will encourage many families to donate who would otherwise not do so.

This long discourse on some of the ethical questions raised by the transplantation of human organs is simply to emphasize that xenotransplantation would eliminate all of the above problems. It would also eliminate the need to use tissues from aborted human fetuses, another source of much controversy and acrimony.

One aspect of the public's attitude to consider is whether there will be any adverse outcome from the *success* of xenotransplantation. After a few well-publicized, even modestly successful xenotransplants in patients, there is a risk that some members of the public will believe that human organs are no longer required. A premature reduction in the donation of cadaveric human organs would, of course, impede the treatment of thousands of patients awaiting transplants.

Another issue to consider is the public's attitude toward a patient who has received a xenotransplant. For example, Jeff Getty, who received baboon cells in an effort to treat his AIDS, has described to us a form of prejudice he calls "human-centrism." Many people, he suggests, believe that xenotransplantation will lead to adulteration of the human species—to the creation of a human-animal. As the recipient of a baboon bone marrow cell transplant, Getty reports being treated as "less than human." He has been introduced in public by the name "baboon boy" (among others), has received gifts of stuffed monkey toys and bananas, and been the victim of endless banana jokes. "Human culture," he said in an interview with the *New York Times* (October 13, 1998), "is full of fascinating mythology about centaurs and werewolves. And I have the feeling that what I've done is touch many people's, including many scientists', deep unconscious fear that xenografting means creating werewolves and monsters." It is unclear whether this fear is real, and, if so, how widespread it may be, or merely perceived. However, as one of the few patients to have received a xenograft, Getty feels this is an important issue that should be addressed. He suggests that it may account for resistance to xenotransplantation on the part of a section of the community.

Risk-Benefit Ratio ∘ ∘ ∘

In Chapter 11 we discussed at some length the potential for the transfer of pathogens from the pig organ to the patient, and also the potential threat to the public health. What will be the community's attitude toward such a risk, when society (as distinct from individuals) will gain no direct benefit from the transplant? The Institute of Medicine committee pointed out that since the general public derives no direct communal benefit, its fear of, and resistance to, xenotransplantation may increase. As in other aspects of xenotransplantation, the role of the media will clearly be important in shaping public opinion in this respect. Although most members of the media may act responsibly, there will no doubt be a few who will sensationalize the risks of infection to the community. If a single xenozoonotic infection does indeed spread from a patient to a close contact, then such reports could generate public hysteria. Xenotransplantation could then come to an abrupt halt.

The benefits and risks of any medical advance have to be carefully weighed using the available facts and expert opinions. A decision to go ahead has to be based on evidence that the benefits appear to outweigh the risks. As the potential benefits to individuals or society increase, it becomes warranted to accept slightly increased risks. Although we have a moral obligation to accept a small risk to the community if the decision leads to great benefits to individuals, we also have an obligation to take all possible steps to minimize the risks to society.

(In the United States, federal regulations require that the degree of risk of an experimental procedure to the patient be "reasonable" in relation to the potential benefit. The benefit can be either to the patient or to society, which will gain from the knowledge obtained. The Institutional Review Board of the hospital where the procedure is to be performed is expected to assess whether the risk-benefit ratio is justified.)

There have, by the way, been many calls from physicians, scientists and others for more public input into the discussion of whether or not xenotransplantation should be advanced into the clinic. The case has been made that, as the health of the community could potentially be at risk, the community itself should decide whether it is willing to accept that risk. There have already been many polls taken to assess public opinion, and numerous meetings held by many government or government-sponsored groups in the United States and the United Kingdom that were either open to the public or which actively sought the opinions of individuals or groups interested in the topic. Furthermore, in most Western countries, the public has been exposed to numerous media presentations on the scientific advances and potential of xenotransplantation. Figures provided by the Imutran press office indicate that in the United Kingdom alone in 1996 there were almost 250 articles in the national press and a further 250 in the regional press. In 1997 there were a further 400 press and magazine articles. The subject was featured on British television or radio approximately 60 times in 1996 and 40 times in 1997. In the United States, more than 400 press pieces were published in 1996, and an estimated 250 more in 1997. In that year, the *New York Times* alone published 24 articles on the topic. Although even more can be done to inform the public of the pros and cons of xenotransplantation—and we hope that this book will contribute in that respect—it is difficult to substantiate a claim that efforts have not been made to do so.

Profit Motives ○ ○ ○

Most, if not all, of us involved with xenotransplantation are influenced to a greater or lesser extent by some form of profit motive. Success for the scientists who develop the transgenic pigs or the drugs that are to be used in the procedure may lead not only to enhancement of professional reputation and academic stature but also to more tangible profits such as improved career opportunities and/or increased financial reward. Moreover, in the past few years, scientists have increasingly been associated directly with biotechnology and pharmaceutical companies as founders, stockholders, employees, or paid consultants, often with stock options. (Both of the authors of this book have financial associations with such companies, as either employee or consultant.) They may therefore have a direct financial interest in the success of their work. Novelist and film director Michael Crichton, himself a Harvard Medical School graduate, has written, "There are no detached observers; nearly every scientist involved in research is also engaged in the commerce of biotechnology."

This association between academia and industry is clearly not a new phenomenon. One has only to look at the development of numerous pieces of medical equipment, such as artificial heart valves or artificial joints. For a number of reasons, however, such associations are more commonplace today than in the past. One reason is the reduction in financial support for medical research available from governmental and charitable institutions. Scientists must often look to industry for the funds in order to continue working in their chosen field. Furthermore, the increasing complexity of medical research requires ever more expensive equipment and facilities to enable it to proceed—as illustrated, for example, by the high cost of developing transgenic livestock.

The surgeons who will perform the surgical procedures may also enhance their reputations. Indeed, to be the first to carry out a successful (or even unsuccessful!) procedure may put a surgeon's name in the history books, and perhaps give him or her a degree of immortality. (One only has to return to Chapter 3 to read the names of several surgeons, now recorded for posterity, who led teams who carried out glaringly unsuccessful xeno-transplants.) The surgeons may directly benefit financially by attracting patients to their surgical practices. If the surgeon also has a direct financial interest in a biotechnology company, this may prove to be another source of pecuniary reward. The commercial companies, whether biotechnology or pharmaceutical, will clearly benefit from the success of their innovations: their stock goes up and they make increased profits.

None of this is new, but the complexity of arrangements between scientists, surgeons, and commercial companies would appear to have increased significantly in recent years, making the financial profit motive a much more significant factor than it has been in the past. All of us are spurred on by one or another profit motive, financial or otherwise, and it would therefore be self-defeating to try to eliminate such motives completely. (The Communist world belatedly arrived at this conclusion about 10 years ago.) However, scientists and surgeons must ensure that this motive does not unduly influence their work or the manner in which the results of their investigations are presented to the scientific community and to the public. If they don't police themselves, then society will be forced to do it for them.

For example, if a biotechnology company is trying to attract investment capital, planning to go public, or attempting to sell itself to a larger company, then there is a risk that the results of its research will be presented to the public in a false light, that is, that the state of the science may be presented as more advanced than it really is. Researchers and surgeons have sought fame and a financially comfortable position for years, but biotechnology companies and investment capitalists are relatively new additions to the scientific community. Commercial interests may therefore begin to influence the scientists' attitude toward publication of their research efforts.

For example, in 1995 a spokesman for one small biotechnology company involved in xenotransplantation announced that the company's technology was "ready for testing in humans." This announcement, by the way, was made to the lay press in the absence of any formal publication of research results in a scientific journal. Soon after—in what was perhaps not a coincidence—the company was purchased by a large pharmaceutical company. The fact that several years have passed since 1995 with no such testing suggests that, for one reason or another, the technology was not ready to be tried in humans. After hearing the announcement, one transplant surgeon with no association with the company said, perhaps with tongue in cheek, that he was "waiting with bated breath" for the clinical trial. Let's hope he is still not holding his breath.

Members of the public are already asking some tough questions. Someone recently posed this question to us: "If a transgenic pig is developed that plays an important role in the success of xenotransplantation, is it ethical for the company that breeds these pigs to make a profit from their sale?" It was clearly the questioner's view that no profit should be derived from this humanitarian enterprise. Human organs are not, after all, bought or sold for profit. Only the essential costs involved in supplying the organ are passed on to the patient or the patient's health care provider, be it private insurance company or government agency.

The question may hinge on whether pig organs should be grouped with human donor organs or with lifesaving devices that, in contrast, have been developed by commercial companies to be sold at a profit. The latter include pig and mechanical heart valves and a multitude of drugs, as well as myriad pieces of equipment ranging from dialysis machines and mechanical cardiac assist devices to intensive care unit monitoring machines. All of these devices save lives, and it is not thought wrong to make a profit from their development and sale. The companies that develop transgenic pigs will expect to make a reasonable profit from their enormous investments of time, money, and resources. This would in no way be considered unethical or unjustified by business standards. The wider financial implications of xenotransplantation to both the patient and community will be discussed more fully in Chapter 16.

Conflicts of Interest:
Who Should Perform the Clinical Trial? o o o

Is it acceptable that those with a direct financial interest (particularly if it involves a major holding of stock) should plan, perform, and report on the initial trial in human patients? Is this ethically optimal? The answer must surely be no. One may also question whether it is even ideal for those performing preclinical studies to be stockholders. Will financial interests influence the manner in which results are presented if venture capital or a boost in the value of the stock is required? Is there a risk that the results of the research will be in some way embellished to reassure existing stockholders and attract new investors? Unfortunately, scientists and doctors are no more immune to such pressures than the rest of society.

Perhaps such animal studies should be performed (or at least confirmed) by a group that is financially independent of the biotechnology company. The benefit to the biotechnology company would be that the results are more likely to be fully accepted by the medical community (just as they are when an independent group of physicians performs a drug trial for a pharmaceutical company). This does not imply that a scientific or medical employee or a paid consultant cannot be directly involved in such studies. Surely, however, there is a conflict of interest if a major stockholder is the principal investigator.

Informed Consent ○ ○ ○

Most Western countries require a patient's consent before performing any clinical research procedure. In the United States, consent is required in both publicly and privately funded research through the Department of Health and Human Services and Food and Drug Administration regulations, respectively. The patient should be given as much information as required to come to a decision whether or not to take part in the research program. The nature and purpose of the research as well as the potential risks (particularly of infection) and benefits to the patient should be explained. With regard to the use of animal organs or tissues, the patient should be given information on the current state of the research, as well as any data relating to the results achieved in patients who have undergone the same, or similar, procedures. This should include the number of deaths, major complications, and the quality of life. Information should also be furnished on any alternative therapies that might be available and on the risks and benefits of these therapies.

As an aside, we call your attention to the enormous strides that have been taken during the past 35 years—partly, it must be admitted, from the fear of malpractice suits—to improve the information that the patient and his or her family receive in order to make an informed decision about a surgical procedure. When the world's first heart transplant—in which a chimpanzee heart was used—was performed by James Hardy in Mississippi in 1964, the consent form signed by the patient's relatives (the patient was semicomatose) consisted of a single paragraph. Although the form did include the statement that no previous heart transplant had ever been performed in a human, there was no mention of the possibility of using a chimpanzee as the donor. There were no indications of possible complications or risks from the operation. We call these points to your attention not to criticize the surgical team or the transplant center, as this was the norm at the time. We wish solely to compare what was legally and morally required little more than 35 years ago with the far more comprehensive efforts that are expected today.

The Baby Fae case in 1984 prompted questions about the ethics of research in human subjects. In particular, there were concerns about how adequate informed consent could be obtained under life-and-death circumstances, especially when a child is involved. For example, the permission form signed by the parents of Baby Fae stated that "this research is an effort to provide your baby with some hope of immediate and long-term survival." Although this truthfully reflected the surgical team's hopes, it was perhaps unduly optimistic for the science of the time.

It has been said that, by today's standards, the behavior of many of the early surgeons and transplant centers who attempted xenotransplantation would be considered unethical. But this serves only to indicate how standards have changed, as they have in many other aspects of our society.

Today, genuine attempts are being made to provide patients and their families all the information they need to give a truly informed consent to any surgical procedure. However, there are some who believe that current methods of obtaining informed consent are inadequate and could be significantly improved. In truth, it is difficult to present a highly complex subject, particularly in the early stages of its development, to patients and expect them to fully comprehend what they are agreeing to, and there are those who question whether informed consent can ever really be obtained with regard to a subject as complex as xenotransplantation. When extremely ill patients are being offered such an option, it is even more difficult for them and their families to weigh the pros and cons.

With regard to the use of animal organs and tissues, it should be stressed to the initial patients that they will be participating in a clinical *experiment*, and that although the experiment may not have a high chance of long-term success, the scientific community hopes and expects to learn a great deal. It may be difficult for many physicians or surgeons, particularly those with any form of personal investment (financial or otherwise) in the performance of the trial, to emphasize this point clearly. Inevitably, surgeons attempt to offer hope to the patient that he or she will benefit directly from the procedure (usually in the form of a prolonged period of good health). Indeed, this may prove to be the case, as with a small handful of the patients who underwent human organ transplantation when it was in its infancy. Those patients, unfortunately, will almost certainly be in the minority. Most subjects will undergo the procedure, possibly survive for a varying but relatively short period of time, and then die from some complication. Their willingness to participate in the trial will have provided the research team with valuable experience and information that will undoubtedly benefit future patients. By the terms of the Declaration of Helsinki, which records the World Medical Association guidelines on research involving human subjects, it is perfectly ethical to carry out an experimental procedure on a patient who has given his or her informed consent, even if the procedure carries some risk for the patient. The declaration has also been interpreted as indicating that such an experiment is justified even if the individual patient is unlikely to benefit personally, as long as future patients with the same underlying problem may benefit. Immunologist Jeff Platt has drawn attention to a patient's right to participate in such a trial by asking, "Is it ethical to deny a patient, especially one dying of some dreadful illness, the satisfaction of serving humanity?"

No matter how enthusiastic a group of researchers is to advance the science, and no matter what the potential benefits may be to future patients, it remains morally reprehensible not to give the individual patient as honest and realistic a picture as possible of the potential benefits and risks. A good argument can be made, therefore, for patient consent to be obtained by an individual who is totally independent of the transplant team—preferably, of course, a physician with knowledge of the field. This individual, who would in no way be involved in the research program, could give valuable counseling to both patient and family, not only about the potential outcome and ramifications of a xenotransplant but also about other possible therapeutic options. University of Texas ethicist Harold Vanderpool, however, believes that this "distrust-driven policy" would possibly prevent the surgical team and the patient from openly discussing the "multifaceted human dimensions" of xenotransplantation. Informed consent has been likened to buying automobile insurance. It is almost impossible for the purchaser to understand all of the minutiae in the contract he is about to sign, and to a large extent he bases his decision on whether he trusts the agent and the insurance company. Granting consent to go ahead with something as complex as a xenotransplant may boil down to a matter of trust between patient and surgeon. However, it would certainly seem beneficial for the patient to have the support of a patient advocate at the time consent is being discussed and requested. It would almost certainly also be valuable to the patient to have the opportunity to discuss what he or she is about to consent to with others who have been through the same or a similar clinical research procedure.

If there is deemed to be any potential risk of the transfer of infection to family members and friends of the patients, it may prove necessary—and certainly wise—to obtain their consent also. Vanderpool has pointed out that such consent would serve as a way to protect xenotransplant researchers and centers from potential legal action. He also draws attention to the U.S. Public Health Service draft guidelines recommending that baseline blood samples be taken from all medical personnel dealing with patients and/or animal organs or cells. These samples are to be stored and are subject to surveillance by U.S. federal agencies. "Should not the consent of these medical workers be requested after they are told who will have access to their test results?"

Vanderpool asks. "And what will happen if serum tests reveal that they have a problematic or embarrassing infection?" The legal repercussions are clearly considerable.

Patient Confidentiality ○ ○ ○

One final point that has not received much attention in the various discussions that have taken place regarding the advance of xenotransplantation from the laboratory into the hospital is the matter of patient confidentiality. The privacy of the patient, and particularly the confidentiality of his or her identity, has been a cornerstone of medical practice, and particularly of all clinical trials, for generations. With a topic that will clearly generate enormous media and public interest, it will undoubtedly prove increasingly difficult to maintain that confidentiality if that is what the patient and his/her family request. There is bound to be competition between representatives of the media for details of the experiences of the first few patients whose lives depend on the performance of newly transplanted pig kidneys or hearts. Leaks will be obtained without difficulty, whether they come from hospital personnel, family members, or neighbors, particularly if the price is right. It is quite conceivable that less reputable members of the media will directly or indirectly reveal details that the patient had requested be kept confidential.

It may be, however, that the patient (and/or the patient's family) will see this opportunity as a final chance for establishing financial security. The personal story of any of the first few patients to be entered into a clinical trial of xenotransplantation will be worth a considerable sum to the media. Bidding wars will break out over this rare commodity. Even if those performing the trial attempt to control the commercial sequelae of the xenotransplant procedure, the determined patient—encouraged, aided, and abetted by ingenious agents and/or lawyers—will find ways to reap maximal financial reward from the unfortunate cards life has dealt him or her. And those of us to whom life has been kinder are possibly in no position to make a judgment on such a patient's decision.

chapter 14

Protecting the Public

Government regulations and safeguards

The Need for Regulations and Safeguards ○ ○ ○

Today, with media attention and the public eye increasingly upon the medical profession—and with the prevailing medico-legal environment—few would disagree that some form of monitoring of clinical trials of xenotransplantation will be essential. Only by a thorough review of the proposed trial, and by its careful monitoring, will we be able to ensure that a "cowboy" approach to xenotransplantation does not prevail—such as occurred after the first human heart transplant in the late 1960s. At that time, numerous inadequately prepared surgical groups rushed into this field without the necessary expertise or laboratory experience. Their results were generally poor and at times disastrous. This led to what essentially constituted a moratorium on heart transplantation for over a decade.

The need for regulation is even greater with regard to xenotransplantation in view of the potential risks. This presents a scenario that is very different from most operative procedures and from the usual drug and device development, which generally present risks only to the patient.

Today, there are basically two distinct types of regulatory bodies charged with overseeing the transfer of xenotransplantation technologies into the realm of patient care. The first is government agencies charged with ensuring the public safety, such as the Food and Drug Administration (FDA) in the United States. A company wishing to introduce a new product or device—be it a specially bred pig, a new drug, or even use of an existing drug for a new purpose, such as xenotransplantation—must obtain the FDA's permission to do so. Once the FDA has approved the product or device, physicians throughout the country are at liberty to prescribe it or use it for the purposes for which it has been approved.

Until the FDA has approved the use of a new drug, device, or biological product, the physician will also be required to obtain the consent of a second body, the ethics committee of the hospital in which the product or procedure is to be used. These hospital committees are responsible for reviewing and agreeing to all proposed clinical research protocols. In the United States, they are known as Institutional Review Boards (IRBs). (There are also Institutional Animal Care and Use Committees (IACUCs), which fulfill the same role with regard to research involving animals, and which would be responsible for ensuring the humane care of the donor animals used in clinical xenotransplantation. Evidence that IACUCs do their job effectively is provided by the fact that in the early 1990s, when surgeons at Columbia Presbyterian Medical Center in New York were considering using a chimpanzee heart to bridge a patient until a human heart could be obtained, it was the IACUC rather than the IRB that declined to approve the plan. The IRB concluded that the proposal was in the patient's best interests, but the IACUC decided that it was not in the best interests of chimpanzees, largely on the grounds that they are an endangered species.)

However, despite the advent of these IRBs, there is still a risk that the chaotic situation of the late 1960s could be repeated today. If one enterprising group achieves a modicum of success in a handful of patients, the likelihood is that numerous other groups with no or little background in organ xenotransplantation will immediately wish to jump on the bandwagon. Even potential medico-legal consequences will not deter some of them. Without some form of regulation, many patients could be subjected to experimentation by groups without sufficient expertise or experience.

Discussions regarding the need for regulation of xenotransplantation have been under way in the United Kingdom and the United States since 1995 (see Appendix). How much regulation there should be and who should do the monitoring remain controversial topics, and until recently, there appeared to be some discrepancy between the views held on either side of the Atlantic.

Who Should Do the Monitoring? o o o

In the United States, the Public Health Service (PHS) of the Department of Health and Human Services (DHHS) drew up draft guidelines in 1996 that likely will have to be followed closely by most (but perhaps not all) teams planning to use animal cells or organs in patients. Adherence to the guidelines will be mandatory for any hospital or organization that receives any federal financial support and for any commercial company. If the xenotransplantation procedure is to be funded entirely from private sources, such as a charity or clinic that receives absolutely no federal funding (which is rare today), then the guidelines may possibly not need to be followed, although this would certainly put the organization at greater legal risk should anything untoward take place.

The guidelines being finalized at present by the U.S. government and its agencies (which we shall review later) are both comprehensive and detailed. Nevertheless, until very recently it appeared that responsibility for adherence to the PHS guidelines would fall primarily on the local medical center where the trial is to be carried out. It was also the conclusion of the 1995 Institute of Medicine committee that guidelines should be formulated, and that the responsibility for the clinical trial itself should be left to the local hospital review committee, the IRB. The DHHS would presumably have enough "muscle" to punish any center that failed to follow these guidelines. This plan is likely to change, as the PHS has subsequently proposed the formation of a National Advisory Committee to oversee xenotransplantation.

The setting up of a national committee to regulate and monitor specific medical research in patients would not be unique. For example, in the United States the Recombinant DNA Advisory Committee was appointed by the National Institutes of Health (NIH) to oversee clinical trials of gene therapy. There is a similar committee in the United Kingdom, the Gene Therapy Advisory Committee. (Gene therapy involves the introduction of genes into cells of the body via specially selected benign viruses. There was concern that under certain circumstances, these "tame" carrier viruses could cause disease in the patient—and perhaps be spread to other members of the community.)

From the outset, U.S. opinion differed from that in the United Kingdom, where the Advisory Group on the Ethics of Xenotransplantation issued a report at the end of 1996 that came down quite firmly on the side of governmental regulation and monitoring. It recommended the establishment of a National Standing Committee (NSC) to "have overall national responsibility" to oversee all aspects of the development of xenotransplantation. The NSC would be responsible for approving all clinical investigations that use xenograft products. The report further recommended that the NSC be established by law, that "a comprehensive statutory framework of regulation be put in place," and that the NSC "should be funded by, and be under the aegis of, the appropriate U.K. Government Departments." The local committees in the United Kingdom, known as the Local Research Ethics Committees, would also have to give approval for any clinical trial, but only after approval had already been given by the NSC.

The NSC has not yet been established, but a Xenotransplantation Interim Regulatory Authority (UKXIRA) has been functioning for more than a year. The British Ministry of Health recently issued a circular to British hospitals in regard to the application requirements for any group wishing to initiate clinical trials of xenotransplantation. Each application will be scrutinized by the UKXIRA (and a panel of expert assessors), which will then advise the minister, who will make the final decision. The use of great apes as source animals will not be allowed, and applications to use other nonhuman primates are unlikely to be granted. (In 1999, perhaps rather belatedly, the DHHS announced the same virtual ban on the use of nonhuman primates in the United States.) Other aspects of the U.K. policy include plans to ensure the welfare of the source animals and a code of practice with regard to the level of biosecurity required in maintaining the animals. The ministry hinted strongly that studies that were not related to therapy of a patient (that is, experiments on volunteers who would not directly benefit from the procedure) would not be permitted. Nor would any procedure be allowed where the patient was not in a position to give his or her informed consent; presumably this would exclude children, patients in a coma, and mentally disabled or disturbed patients.

Central control may be seen to be preferable in the United Kingdom possibly because xenotransplantation will be carried out within a government-financed, socialized national health service. However, the U.K. Advisory Group considered the possibility that clinical trials might take place in the private sector of the health care community (that is to say, at a medical facility outside of the government-financed National Health Service) and therefore might not fall under the control of the proposed NSC. The advisory group recommended that the "approval of the NSC should be regarded as a condition for obtaining registration (or remaining registered) under Part II of the Registered Homes Act 1984." The implied threat is that authorization to continue as a provider of medical care would not be renewed if a private institution allowed xenotransplantation to proceed without NSC approval.

Which of these two policies—local control, as originally recommended in the United States, or central control, as envisaged in the United Kingdom—is the right one? Can a local committee, even with the help of detailed PHS guidelines, adequately perform the role expected of it? Possibly—but probably not. Local committees, such as the IRB, are made up primarily of local physicians, but also include other members of the community. There is usually at least one nonscientist and one member representing the community who is not associated with the institution in any way. Such a group rarely has expertise in cutting-edge research such as gene therapy or xenotransplantation. Although members of hospital IRBs are frequently inadequately informed about the science involved in a new field, one could argue that they do not need to know much about the science, as their main task is to consider the ethics. Without a solid scientific foundation, however, it is surely difficult, if not impossible, to make an informed ethical decision. Furthermore, some hospital IRBs are susceptible (consciously or unconsciously) to persuasion or manipulation by dominant personalities, who may include those seeking IRB approval. If the only expert is the physician or surgeon seeking permission to pursue the clinical trial, he or she can at times unduly influence those less well informed. The major problem with any committee that does not include recognized experts is that, to a large extent, it has to accept the information given to it by the proposers of the trial. Yet if it receives only selected information, there is a likelihood that its decision will be erroneous.

It would seem that only a regional, national, or even international committee will contain sufficient expertise and knowledge to adequately assess a proposed clinical trial. Such a committee would act as a peer review body for those proposing the trial. Members would include experts in the field of clinical organ transplantation, experimental xenotransplantation, microbiology, genetic engineering, veterinary medicine, and so on, as well as nonscientists. The committee's comprehensive knowledge of the field would ensure that (i) no other acceptable form of therapy is likely to succeed or is available to the patient at the appropriate time; (ii) the necessary laboratory studies have been performed before the group carries out the clinical trial; (iii) the investigators have the necessary expertise to perform such a trial; (iv) the trial is well planned and is likely to provide a definitive answer; (v) the animals being used will be treated humanely; (vi) the necessary safeguards have been taken, for example, with regard to excluding transfer of viral pathogens with the transplanted organ; (vii) truly informed consent has been obtained, possibly by insisting that an independent physician obtains this consent rather than a member of the surgical team; and (viii) there is no undue influence from any profit motive. Furthermore, the committee may wish to ensure that the trial, unless part of a multicenter study, is not being duplicated elsewhere, thereby risking unnecessary suffering and expense. In fact, this arrangement would also benefit the local surgical team. Not only would the committee share responsibility for the trial, but any subsequent criticism of the trial (or unanticipated adverse complications) could be referred back to the committee, whose members would be expected to defend their decision to allow the trial to proceed. The choice of government agency to oversee such a committee—the FDA or the NIH in the United States (or their equivalents in other countries)—would be less important than the fact that such a committee exists and that all centers planning clinical trials would be allowed to proceed only with the consent of the committee.

The arguments against the establishment of such a committee, particularly one with the power to prevent or postpone a planned clinical trial, are several. One is the fear that it might become an elite group that tries to confine research to a select few centers, thus impeding new approaches by those on the "outside." However, this does not appear to have happened in the case of the Recombinant DNA Advisory Committee. A second argument points to the delays and red tape possible with such bureaucracy. Although these are certainly risks with any such system, they are not inevitable. The relatively speedy decision by the FDA to allow transplantation of baboon bone marrow into a patient with AIDS (despite considerable expert advice against it) provides support for this belief. However, even if some delay occurs, the risk to patients—and, in view of the potential for spread of infection, possibly to the community—surely justifies such an ordered, supervised approach. It is a small price to have to pay.

What Regulations Are Necessary? o o o

Most of the regulations in xenotransplantation relate to the risk of transmitting infectious diseases. This topic was clearly paramount in the eyes of the Institute of Medicine, as it was with the PHS. The institute recommended the establishment of guidelines to (i) screen source animals for infectious organisms; (ii) monitor xenotransplant patients throughout their lifetimes and periodically monitor persons with whom they come into contact (families, health care workers, and so on) for evidence of infectious disease; (iii) store tissue and blood samples (which may prove valuable for retrospective study if the patient shows signs of infection or when new diagnostic tests become available) from both the source animals and human recipients; and (iv) maintain national and local registries of patients receiving xenotransplants. Other bodies have suggested additional regulatory safeguards, including such matters as registration of those involved in the breeding and supply of the donor animals, and the tracking and controlling of the geographic disposal of donor tissues. It is also likely the guidelines will call for counseling of xenograft recipients, informing them that they should not donate blood or organs. Informed consent, both of the risks and of the possible need for monitoring the patient's partners, will also be required.

The PHS is clearly taking the potential risks seriously. Consider, for example, the immense amount of work involved in monitoring all of the animals, the patients, and those who have contact with either animals or patients. The perceptive reader of these guidelines, which relate to a procedure with only a *potential* risk to the community, may quickly conclude that they are far stricter than those that pertain to a patient with AIDS, for example, who is a *known* risk to other members of the community. This reflects the fact that xenotransplantation will be introduced purposely as a clinical experiment, whereas AIDS is considered an experiment of nature and therefore not subject to the same regulation. The British and now the American authorities are envisaging national xenotransplantation registry databases to collect data on all of the early patients who undergo xenotransplantation. This caution on the part of the health authorities almost certainly reflects the sobering experience gained in recent years from AIDS and other conditions, such as "mad cow" disease. It would seem that they are determined not to be caught by surprise again.

There is, of course, one more important factor in this equation. Xenotransplantation will inevitably involve the introduction of a new "product," namely, the specially bred, defined-pathogen-free donor pig. The pig must therefore pass the rigorous tests required of any new product. The demands put on manufacturers who plan to sell a product are, in general, much greater than those placed on physicians or institutions treating diseases.

Furthermore, in recent years, we have become acutely aware of the potential risks of the transfer of infection through something as benign-seeming as a blood transfusion. Tragically, viruses such as those that cause AIDS and hepatitis have been passed on by this route. Would blood transfusions—which can be counted in their millions each year—be introduced today, now that the potential risks are known? Indeed, would the transplantation of human organs, which can also transfer infection, be accepted by the authorities today? Both blood transfusion and organ transplantation provide good examples of how the medical profession, representing society in general, has been faced with determining the relative risk-benefit ratio of a procedure. Xenotransplantation will require its own risk-benefit ratio to be determined. If this ratio is as good as those of blood transfusion and human organ transplantation, it too will be accepted.

The PHS guidelines address several specific points. Significantly, they recommend archiving of tissues from the donor pig for 50 years, and they suggest the patient undergo surveillance for life. How far a person's privacy can be invaded in an effort to monitor his or her lifestyle and human contacts may prove controversial. Such an intrusion, particularly into one's sexual life, could prove intolerable even to a hitherto stable individual. As we have noted, this is one of the reasons great care will be required in the selection of the first few patients. A thorough psychological assessment may help to ensure that they are likely to both comply with and tolerate the extraordinary demands that will be made upon them for the rest of their lives.

True, organ transplant patients are already monitored by their doctors for life—but not to the degree that is envisaged with regard to the first xenotransplant patients. Furthermore, transplant recipients sometimes become less compliant once the initial few post-transplant months have progressed successfully. We have known patients with heart transplants who, for one reason or another, have persistently failed to attend follow-up clinics. Some have failed to take their immunosuppressive medication regularly, or have reverted to heavy smoking or alcohol intake against their physician's advice. Others have failed to report infections when these have developed. Several of these patients have died as a direct result of their noncompliance.

This can be for a number of reasons. Depression brought on by the patient's medical or social condition, for example, or inability to find a job after a successful transplant is a common cause of such noncompliance. In countries such as the United States, where there is limited socialized medical care, financial problems may be a factor: patients may not be able to afford the very drugs they need to sustain their lives—and so may fail to take them regularly, or they may fail to keep appointments at the hospital for fear of the bill they will receive. Finally, like other human beings, some patients will agree to a commitment when desperate, yet renege on it once they are no longer under the gun.

No matter how carefully patients are screened before they undergo organ xenotransplantation, it is inconceivable that they will all remain compliant with regard to everything that is expected of them under the suggested PHS guidelines. Even if a failure to abide by their initial agreement is made a matter for the courts—an unrealistic prospect—one can foresee a defense, namely that the agreement was signed under duress due to the impending prospect of loss of life. Furthermore, it will clearly be impossible to monitor all of a patient's social and sexual contacts.

These problems were clearly anticipated by the Institute of Medicine committee, which recommended further investigation into the issue of informed consent "in light of the requirement for lifetime surveillance of patients." It concluded that the potential of xenotransplantation is great enough to justify funding of research "necessary to minimize the risk of disease transmission."

What is being envisaged is no longer a simple matter of the patient's signing a consent form after being provided with the necessary information. In view of the perceived potential risk to the community from infection passed from the patient to his or her contacts, the patient will be expected to enter into what can be considered a "contract" with the surgical team and transplant center. Some have suggested that this might have to be a binding legal contract. The patient—and possibly even members of the patient's family—will agree to lifelong monitoring in return for the potential benefits that might result from undergoing the xenotransplant. It must also be remembered that even when the transplant fails—if, say, a transplanted pig kidney is lost from rejection and is removed from the patient's body—the patient, even though now supported by dialysis in this case, will still be required to be monitored for the remainder of his or her life. After death, autopsy would also probably become mandatory. One of the usual features of a patient's consent to participate in a clinical trial is that he or she has the right to withdraw at any time from the experiment. This will presumably no longer be acceptable. Like any contract, however, this one could be broken by one or other party. If the patient reneges on the agreement, the only recourses open to the transplant center would be to cease to provide medical care—which would open a whole new can of ethical worms—or to turn to the law in an attempt to force the patient to comply with the terms of the contract, which would open a different can of worms.

The U.S. PHS draft guidelines propose that the patient should "educate his/her close contacts regarding the possibility of the emergence of xenogeneic infections." Ethicist Harold Vanderpool questions whether this is sufficient. Should not the patient's close contacts also be asked for their informed consent? After all, treatment of the patient will directly affect their lives. For example, they may be recommended to abstain from sexual contact, and may be required to undergo blood tests. But exactly who should be asked to give their consent? If family members, how close must the relationship be? If friends, which ones and how many? Practically, it may boil down to those who are at risk from the exchange of bodily fluids, including semen and saliva.

Surgeon Abdul Daar asks the provocative question "What *would* we do with a recipient and contacts who harbor an unknown or untreatable virus that is spreading rapidly and killing thousands?" In the movie based on Robin Cook's novel *Outbreak,* an African village is deliberately annihilated to prevent the spread of a deadly virus. Daar suggests that in our scenario, it would be seemingly impossible to achieve a degree of quarantine or physical restriction that both protects the public and is compatible with the individual's basic rights. We hope, however, with the identification of this potential problem at this stage, and with the great efforts currently being made—not least by resourceful pharmaceutical companies such as Novartis—to ensure that such a scenario does not occur, we shall never have to answer Daar's spine-chilling question.

The potential for the spread of infection to members of the public—a risk that is not a factor in most other clinical research endeavors—makes the decision to proceed with xenotransplantation one of immense importance. It would seem sensible, therefore, that it be taken only after full consideration of all aspects of the matter by the best experts that the international community can put together. Once the decision has been made, all aspects of the clinical trial must be monitored carefully by the same panel of experts—for several years, if necessary—until it has been confirmed that xenotransplantation provides no hazard to the public health. Virologist Frederick Murphy has stressed that only a national virology laboratory would have the facilities and resources to carry out the monitoring required in the initial patients. In our view, therefore, only a national advisory group, backed by the legal and enforcing powers of government agencies, can satisfactorily perform this supervisory role.

There is one rider to this conclusion. In this age of rapid and easy world travel, a call has been made for any regulations relating to xenotransplantation to be "globalized," a word chosen by Abdul Daar. Just as the Ebola virus could be carried around the world within 24 hours, so there could be a potential risk from the movements of a patient with a xenograft. Daar is concerned that xenotransplantation procedures may be carried out in a country "where the regulations are lax and the scientific base and facilities are inadequate." Although survival of patients in such "xenohavens" may initially be limited, this is a matter that certainly requires international, rather than national, attention and agreement. Amy Patterson of the FDA has pointed out that while the patients may carry passports and go through customs inspections, the microorganisms they carry will not. Others have also emphasized the need to prevent what they have termed "xenotourism."

The governments of several countries—Canada, France, Germany, Spain, Sweden, and the Netherlands, among them—have recently set up advisory committees or commissions to advise them on the implications of xenotransplantation and the steps that need to be taken to protect both the patient and the public health. Indeed, Spain can lay claim to being the first country to actually publish official guidelines for the procedure (see *Nature*

Medicine 4, 876, 1998). The Council of Europe, representing 40 countries, released a recommendation on xenotransplantation that was adopted by the Committee of Ministers in 1997. However, in 1999 the Council called for a moratorium on clinical trials until the risks of infection to the public have been better assessed. This growing interest in the topic at governmental levels suggests that international agreements will be reached in due course in an attempt to safeguard the public from any potential risks. A recent review and report on the global implications of xenotransplantation by the World Health Organization is an important start. Nonetheless, the power and influence of international agencies is limited in many countries, and the risk of "xeno-tourism," albeit small, will probably always be with us.

To end this chapter on a cautionary note, society has to accept that there will remain some risk. No matter how much government regulation is put in place, no safeguard—short of never attempting to make medical progress—is absolute. To quote Frederick Murphy, "In dealing with infectious diseases, the reality is that our best efforts may decrease but will never eliminate risk." Ultimately, society will have to determine if it is willing to accept this risk.

chapter 15

Judgment Day

Potential legal problems

o o o There has been little consideration of the legal implications of xenotransplantation. Much of the legal literature on organ transplantation focuses on the shortage of human organs and the allocation of these scarce resources to needy patients. In the United States, for example, these matters are covered by the National Organ Transplant Act. The legal issues underlying the shortage of organs will prove largely irrelevant if xenotransplantation becomes a clinical reality, although a host of new legal questions will almost certainly arise.

Sanders Chae, then a young law student who was working with one of us at Harvard, was one of the first to review the potential legal problems that may face us when xenotransplantation advances into the clinic. He considered four major legal issues: whether xenotransplantation is permitted under current law, the potential legal consequences of creating animals with human tissues (and vice versa), the legal aspects of regulating the allocation and distribution of animal organs, and the legal consequences to a transplant center if the public health is put at risk by an infected animal-organ recipient. Although his investigation and conclusions primarily relate to the laws in the United States, they are highly relevant for all Western societies and have implications for all countries where medical science is advanced enough to contemplate xenotransplantation.

Is Xenotransplantation Legally Permissible? ○ ○ ○

In the United States, as in most Western countries, there do not appear to be any laws that specifically prohibit xenotransplantation. In many countries there are laws that explicitly prohibit the sale of human organs, but none that comment on the sale or purchase of animal organs or tissues. Moreover, experimental xenotransplantation is legally permitted in most Western countries, under such legal frameworks as the Animal Welfare Act in the United States. That act attempts to regulate the use of animals in scientific research and requires investigators to provide animals with "humane care and treatment." The breeding of animals for use as donors of organs for humans should be legally acceptable if the animals are bred and housed under similar conditions.

There are also no restrictions on xenotransplantation at common law, which is the system of law in the United States and the United Kingdom that derives its authority from previous judgments and decrees. In most Western countries, judges have at one time or another decided that animals do not have rights under common law. Those decisions act as precedents upon courts today. Without legal rights for animals, no one can bring a lawsuit on behalf of an animal. Additionally, in the United States, animals do not have constitutional rights, such as the right to due process of law.

However, most countries have passed statutes that prohibit cruelty to animals. The legal test of cruelty to an animal is whether the act, omission, or neglect is unjustifiable and causes the animal to experience pain, suffering, or death. The legal standard governing the justifiability of an action toward an animal is that the goal or objective of the action must be reasonable and adequate. Judges have long construed the breeding of animals, such as pigs or cows, for food as a reasonable and adequate goal. They are therefore likely to view the breeding of animals for their organs as equally justifiable. As there are in existence farms housing 300,000 pigs, it is unlikely that a judge could object to a much smaller xenotransplant industry. On the other hand, a court would object to the use of organs from specified animals, such as great apes, that are considered endangered species and are legally protected as such.

The Legal Status of Humans with Animal Parts and Animals with Human Parts ○ ○ ○

Although animals do not have legal rights under common law (at present), creative lawyers supported by animal rights groups will surely attempt to raise novel arguments about the legal status of animals that are to be used in xenotransplantation. Indeed, there are already lawyers in the United States who specialize in protecting (and expanding) the "rights" of animals, particularly household pets. In particular, the prospect of humans with animal organs or transgenic animals that express human genes and have human tissues may blur the distinction between humans and animals. Animal rights groups and other opponents of xenotransplantation might contend that legal rights accompany human tissue and that any being with human cells should possess at least the right to life.

Such arguments may plunge xenotransplantation into a legal gray zone. In most countries, the law has been loath to delineate specifically what constitutes a human being and what does not. This historical reluctance is perhaps understandable, since any definition of a human being is likely to meet with controversy. For example, society is divided about whether fetuses or people in a vegetative coma truly constitute human beings. What constitues a human being will become even more difficult to define now that human cloning is a scientific possibility. If a single cell can be taken from an adult human (who has full legal rights) and a complete human grown from it, then at what stage of development does that cell have legal rights?

The U.S. Congress's recent amendment to the Patent Act is a good example of the law's reluctance to define a human being. Responding to genetic research that has produced transgenic beings expressing both human and animal genes, Congress prohibited the awarding of patents on humans, stating that "human beings are not to be considered patentable subject matter." Congress did not, however, define what a human being is.

A transgenic animal, or even an animal with a human organ, will not enjoy new rights at common law. The law has never recognized legal rights on the basis of human tissue or human cells. Human blood cells or organs are clearly not human beings. A pig with some human cells will still be considered a pig, and likewise, a man who receives an animal organ transplant will not forfeit his legal rights on the operating table.

Some might argue that the law has made tentative steps toward defining a human by human brain activity. In several countries, including the United States, an individual who has sustained total and irreversible loss of brain functioning is legally characterized as dead, and therefore no longer a human being. The 1978 Uniform Brain Death Act in the United States and similar acts in other Western countries were passed in part to help clarify matters relating to the retrieval of human organs for transplantation.

One might extend this rationale and argue that the law considers anyone who enjoys human brain functioning to be a human being and thus entitled to the full panoply of rights. However, this argument is tenuous at best. So little is understood about the human brain, mind, and cognition that any attempt to ground legal rights in the human mind might prove as contested as the notion that the human soul is lodged in the human heart. Moreover, surgeons are already conducting transplants of animal brain cells into the brains of patients with conditions such as Parkinson's disease. Whether future xenotransplants will conceivably affect human mental activity remains speculative. Such transplants, however, could further confound an already confusing subject. Nevertheless, the suggestion that the law recognizes human life according to human brain functioning perhaps offers a tentative standard, at least until neuroscience has developed a better understanding of the relationship between human life and the mind. (On these grounds, however, our concept of human life may be tested in the future by advanced computers with artificial intelligence.)

As an aside, under Dutch law, organs from genetically modified donor animals are covered by legislation that relates to all genetically modified organisms, whether they are pigs or bacteria. This legislation is designed to protect the environment and the public health from any adverse effects from the release of such organisms into the environment. Under this legislation, the human recipient of a transgenic pig organ would come under the scope of the Environmentally Hazardous Substances Act (and would technically be considered a hazard to the environment). A suggestion has been made to exclude such patients from the scope of the act. As pointed out by the committee set up to advise the Dutch government on xenotransplantation, this example suggests that the law as it stands at present is not adequate for regulating biomedical development. This is almost certainly the case in many countries.

Is cannibalism legal?

The question may also arise whether it will be legally permissible, after organ removal, to eat the meat of transgenic animals containing human cells or proteins. It should be remembered that it is not just the donor organs that will contain human proteins or sugars, but also the blood vessels throughout the rest of the body, including the muscles and fat. In other words, bacon and pork chops will also contain human proteins. The consumption of such meat, even though the amount of human protein may be minimal, might be deemed cannibalism. Perhaps surprisingly, there are no legal prohibitions on cannibalism in any U.S. state except Idaho, and we suspect this may be the case in many other countries. The practice in the United States of human "vampires" drinking human blood is certainly not unknown and (outside of Idaho) is not illegal. Even in Idaho, the prohibition applies only to the consumption of tissues or blood from a human being and would thus not apply to meat from transgenic animals. (It should be emphasized, however, that those currently in the business of developing herds of transgenic pigs have no intention of making the meat available for consumption by humans or any other animal species.)

How Should Animal Organs Be Distributed? o o o

Because of the chronic shortage of human organs, many countries have passed acts relating to organ donation and transplantation. In the United States, for example, the National Organ Transplant Act created a centralized system called the Organ Procurement and Transplant Network (OPTN). A national computer registry was also set up; this matches available organs to potential recipients on the basis of medical criteria, such as urgency and tissue compatibility. The United Network for Organ Sharing (UNOS) administers the OPTN and the national transplant registry. Other Western countries (or groups of countries) have similar organizations, such as U.K. Transplant, France Transplant, and Eurotransplant.

Successful xenotransplantation would eliminate the shortage of organs and would call into question whether such a central service is the most effective way to distribute organs. Governments could either maintain a centralized system or permit a commercial system based on market forces. If a central service were retained, centers that breed donor animals would be required to supply the organs to patients through the central distribution system. Attempts to sell animal organs outside of the system would presumably be illegal, just as the sale or purchase of human organs today is illegal.

However, governments might not find animal organs sufficiently different from other health care products, such as artificial or animal heart valves, to justify centralized regulation. Market forces already influence most facets of medical treatment, particularly in the United States. If a government permitted such commercial systems, legal regulation of the animal breeding and transplant centers as commercial entities would be limited to issues such as licensing requirements. The only remaining role for a centralized service would be the monitoring of xenotransplantation activity by the maintenance of a national registry. This would assess the success of xenotransplantation and track the potential transmission of infectious diseases.

But would the introduction of a market-driven distribution of animal organs function satisfactorily alongside a centralized controlled system of distributing human organs? Or would there be pressure to distribute human organs by the same market forces? (A strong case for a market-driven system for human organs, whether or not xenotransplantation becomes a reality, has been made by lawyer and economist Lloyd Cohen, of George Mason University in Virginia. His argument that "if you pay people for something, they will provide more of it than if you do not" is highly persuasive, if controversial.) If human organs were sold and purchased, and if human organs were demonstrated to result in longer survival than when a pig organ is transplanted (as is initially likely), then the price of human organs might be pushed higher and higher. Clearly, these potential problems need to be addressed before clinical xenotransplantation is introduced, and legal measures must be taken to prevent them from occurring.

The Legal Consequences of Endangering the Public Health ○ ○ ○

At present, there are no laws that specifically govern xenotransplantation. In most countries, however, there exist legal frameworks that could grant authority to the government (or government agencies) to regulate this form of therapy, particularly to diminish the risk of the spread of infectious disease. For example, genetically modified pig organs will presumably require some form of quality control that will be overseen by a government agency, such as the Food and Drug Administration (FDA) in the United States. But if this system of approval fails, there are other legal routes by which xenotransplantation could be controlled. As an example, let us examine the legal situation in the United States.

First, there are already laws that would grant the Public Health Service (PHS), the Department of Health and Human Services (DHHS), and the FDA the power to regulate animal organs, tissues, and cells as "biological products." Selling, bartering, or exchanging a biological product is prohibited unless it was prepared at an establishment licensed by the DHSS. To qualify for a license, a facility must comply with PHS standards and guidelines. Centers will therefore have to comply with current and future PHS guidelines before they can obtain a DHHS license to breed animals for their organs. More significant is that the PHS has the authority to remove biological products from the market if these threaten the public health and safety. Thus, the PHS has the power not only to regulate xenotransplantation centers but also to shut them down if the potential for infectious disease poses a risk to the public.

Second, the DHSS and the FDA may have the legal authority to regulate animal organs as "devices." The category of "devices" is not limited only to man-made or artificial implants; it also includes live tissue grafts. The DHSS and the FDA are empowered to ban devices that threaten public health and safety. Furthermore, the Medical Research Modernization Committee drew attention to the point that clinical trials of xenotransplantation could violate the National Environmental Policy Act. This mandates that federal agencies have to prepare environmental impact statements before allowing the use of a technology that could adversely impact the human environment (by, for example, exposing the public to novel infections). This would provide a justification for removing animal organs from the market if need be.

A transplant center could also be liable in a lawsuit for having committed a tort—that is to say, for a civil wrong done against another person for which the law will recompense the victim. Medical malpractice, for example, is a tort. In a situation where an infectious disease has been transmitted, there are several types of actions that could lead to lawsuits against the transplant center.

The basic tort lawsuit is a negligence action. Negligence is defined as conduct that imposes an unreasonable risk upon others. The plaintiff must prove that the defendant owed a legal duty to avoid creating unreasonable risks, that the defendant breached that legal duty, that the breach has caused the plaintiff an injury, and that he or she has suffered actual damage from the breach.

Two negligence actions could be raised. First, a transplant patient who contracts a known or unknown infectious disease could raise a tort suit against the transplant surgeon and the center. Both doctor and center, of course, have a duty to their patient to act reasonably. However, there is no issue of malpractice if the center and surgeon have complied with relevant regulations and standards of medical conduct. Such a lawsuit would be on weak ground because the patient will presumably have consented to the procedure with knowledge of the risks involved. If the patient was given an accurate and comprehensible warning of the risks before the procedure, the common law considers the patient to have made an "assumption of risk" and will reject a negligence suit.

The other potential plaintiff is a member of the general public who contracts an infectious disease from a patient with an animal organ transplant. Those most at risk would be the patient's family and friends, as well as medical, nursing, and paramedical staff who had contact with the patient. It could be argued that such persons were aware of the risks of contact with the patient and had made an "assumption of risk" themselves. (It should not be forgotten that many of the early liver and kidney transplant surgeons and nurses contracted hepatitis from their patients. Several became very ill, and some actually died.) Thus, the most likely plaintiff to succeed in such a suit would be an individual who was unaware of the risks of close contact with the patient. If the transferred infection is a known and treatable one, and the transplant patient failed to make every reasonable effort to limit exposure of other individuals to the disease, then the plaintiff could sue the patient for being negligent and could seek financial compensation.

A more complicated case arises if the transmitted disease was hitherto unknown or untreatable. In that event, there may be little that the transplant patient could have done to limit the public's exposure to the disease. However, a court might find that the transplant hospital owes a legal duty to the public not to introduce infectious diseases into the public domain. The performance of xenotransplantation could be ruled a breach of that duty. The outcome of such a case would to some extent depend on how a jury balances the potential benefit of xenotransplantation to the patient and to society against the risk of releasing a previously unknown xenozoonosis into the general public. How closely the transplant institution had followed the PHS guidelines would also clearly be important.

A second type of tort suit is the claim that the transplant center carried out an "ultrahazardous" or "abnormally dangerous" activity. There are, as one might expect, legal variations in what constitutes such activity. An ultrahazardous activity is defined as one that necessarily involves a risk of serious harm to the person, land, or chattels of others, cannot be eliminated by the exercise of utmost care, and is not a matter of common usage. An abnormally dangerous activity is, in addition, inappropriate to the place where it is carried on, and one whose value to the community is outweighed by its dangerous attributes.

The typical case arises from blasting, crop dusting, or spraying, the storage and transport of toxic chemicals and flammable liquids, or from the use and storage of explosives. However, an inventive lawyer could attempt to include animal organ transplants within the definition, particularly in light of the opinion of its potential risks published by virologists and other infectious-disease experts. Grafting an animal organ into a human recipient is not a matter of common usage, and the transmission of an unknown xenozoonosis is a serious harm that could not be eliminated by the exercise of utmost care. However, the activity might be considered appropriate to where it is carried out (a transplant center), and the benefits to the patient and society might outweigh the potential risk of harm.

A transplant center could also be sued for having created a public nuisance. For more than a century, U.S. common law has recognized interferences with the public health as a public nuisance—not only through the possible transmission of an infectious disease but, for example, through the keeping of disease-ridden animals. The usual consequence for having committed a public nuisance is that the community, the state, or representatives of the community are entitled to stop the defendant from continuing to create the nuisance. Hence, a transplant center in the United States could be shut down even if the DHHS or PHS has permitted it to perform xenotransplantation. The public nuisance tort effectively creates a separate standard that transplant hospitals must meet in addition to the explicit requirements that they must satisfy to procure an operating license.

Tort liability will be an important issue in xenotransplantation. It could cripple the industry, despite the significant benefits that xenotransplantation might offer. One possible solution suggested by Sanders Chae might be the introduction of a no-fault insurance program. Consider, for example, the National Vaccine Injury Compensation Program in the United States. Any individual who has suffered an illness or death from receiving a vaccine, or any individual who has contracted polio from a recipient of the polio vaccine, may file a petition for compensation without the need to demonstrate negligence or fault by the manufacturer. However, financial compensation is limited, and punitive damages are not awarded. Victims therefore have the option either to bring a petition under the no-fault standard or to bring a civil lawsuit in state court. The latter, however, requires a much higher standard of proof. The U.S. Congress established such a system to protect vaccine manufacturers against tort suits that threatened to bankrupt the industry. Given the significant potential benefits that xenotransplantation presents, a comparable program that would compensate victims who contract a xenozoonosis could limit potential tort liability.

The above examples indicate that, as with most advances in biotechnology, xenotransplantation may challenge society with difficult ethical and legal questions. Legal decisions and the introduction of new laws will be influenced by the public attitude toward this form of therapy, and will depend to a great degree on whether society embraces it wholeheartedly or not.

chapter 16

The Ultimate Piggy Bank

Animal transplants and health care economics

Making a Buck:
The Financial Impact of Xenotransplantation o o o

When the first tentative reports on the use of pig brain cells in the treatment of patients with Parkinson's disease reached the public in 1995, Dr. Philip Noguchi, the FDA physician overseeing the regulation of xenotransplantation, received telephone calls from pig farmers inquiring how they could get involved in what they perceived as a potentially profitable commercial venture. This anecdote exemplifies the universal wish to "make a buck," no matter what the venture. However, given the very strict requirements for the breeding and housing of the pigs to be used in xenotransplantation, the average hog farmer is unlikely to reap any financial reward from xenotransplantation. Many others undoubtedly will.

Successful xenotransplantation will clearly have a major financial impact on health care; the effects will be felt both by the community and by the individual patient. Its impact is difficult to predict in detail, as there will be both savings and increased expenditure. Money will be saved on such items as long-term dialysis, which will no longer be necessary in the majority of kidney patients, but dollars will be expended on the much larger number of organ transplants that will be performed. Nonetheless, xenotransplantation's overall impact on national health care economics will almost certainly be to engender considerably increased expenditure. Whenever money is spent, from whatever source, there are those who have to foot the bill, in this case either government or insurance companies. But, of course, there are also those who benefit financially, for example, transplant centers and surgeons, transgenic pig breeders, and pharmaceutical companies.

Even with the increasing use of organs from living human donors (usually relatives of the recipient, and largely restricted to kidneys and partial liver grafts), the amount spent on transplantation remains predominantly restricted by the shortage of cadaveric donor organs. Without a donor organ, there can be no transplant. With successful xenotransplantation, the number of organs will be unlimited, and there will no longer be any such restriction. Not only will all patients on the waiting list be able to undergo an organ transplant immediately, but many borderline candidates, currently *not* on the waiting list, will also have a chance for a better life. Furthermore, transplantation will become available to patients in countries such as Japan, where cadaveric organ donation, although now legal, is not yet fully accepted culturally. The number of organ transplants being performed worldwide may well immediately double, and continue to grow each year. Our experience is that once a form of therapy is proven and becomes established, suitable candidates begin to come out of the woodwork and the number of patients seeking such therapy expands rapidly.

According to a 1996 report by Salomon Brothers, a leading London investment banking house, the annual number of organ transplants is expected to rise from approximately 45,000 worldwide today to between 300,000 and 500,000 by the year 2010. The time scale of this prediction is already probably inaccurate, for it is extremely unlikely that xenotransplantation will have developed to the extent that such large numbers of transplants can be performed by 2010. Nevertheless, the detailed observations and calculations made in producing this report give some idea of the impact that xenotransplantation may make. Certainly, the 20,000 organ transplants performed in the United States each year are likely to increase to at least 50,000 to 100,000. The impact of cell xenotransplants on the treatment of diabetics may be huge, with many thousands of patients undergoing islet cell engraftment each year. If other conditions such as Parkinson's and Alzheimer's diseases prove amenable to therapy by cell transplantation, then xenotransplantation procedures may be carried out in the hundreds of thousands every year.

The Economics of Transplantation:
Health Care Dollars and Sense ○ ○ ○

One of the few economists who has made an independent study of the economics of organ transplantation is Roger Evans, a professor in the Department of Health Sciences Research and head of the Section of Health Service Education at the Mayo Clinic in Minnesota. Evans has studied the financial aspects of organ transplantation in the United States for over 20 years. He estimates the annual amount of health care dollars spent on patients with organ transplants in the United States today exceeds $5 billion. (David Harper, chief scientist of the United Kingdom's Department of Health, puts worldwide expenditure on transplantation at double this amount.) Although this is a considerable sum of money, it represents less than 0.5% of the total health care budget of the United States, which now exceeds $1 trillion annually. These estimates are based on the actual amounts billed to insurance companies and other payors. It is usual, however, for the providers of health care—hospitals, physicians, allied professionals—to be reimbursed less than they bill. This is because many health insurance policies, including the government-sponsored Medicare program (which covers the cost of the majority of kidney transplants performed in the United States), limit payment on various services. The providers have therefore become accustomed to receiving less than they ask for. The amount actually spent on organ transplantation is therefore probably rather less than the figure given above.

The expenditure on transplantation (and, indeed, on all other procedures) may actually decrease in the United States during the next few years as more and more patients fall under the umbrella of managed care. Health insurance providers and health maintenance organizations, known as HMOs, are increasingly negotiating flat rates for particular therapeutic procedures, such as organ transplants. The insurer and the provider negotiate a set fee to be paid to the hospital and/or physician for a specific organ transplant performed in a single patient, for example, a patient undergoing heart transplantation. This fee covers all aspects of the patient's care, including the expenses associated with retrieval of the donor organ, the operation itself (often including the fee of the surgeon and his team), the postoperative in-hospital care, the cost of immunosuppressive drugs, and all follow-up for the first post-transplant year. The transplant center knows what it will be paid and can therefore budget accordingly, and the insurer has a guarantee that the costs incurred will be strictly limited.

Such a system puts great pressure on the transplant center to keep its costs to a minimum, and to some extent it helps to curtail the escalating cost of health insurance to the individual. If the transplant center can restrict its expenditure to less than the fee it will receive, then it will make a profit. However, if the patient develops complications that necessitate a prolonged hospital stay—particularly if in the intensive care unit—or repeated readmissions, then the transplant center will lose money on the deal. (A similar system now exists in the United Kingdom, where the payor, in this case usually the patient's primary-care physician, negotiates a contract with the hospital providing the service, even though all of the funds are ultimately made available through the government-funded national health service.)

Roger Evans estimates that if the number of such contracts negotiated between insurer and transplant center continues to rise, the amount spent on organ transplantation annually may actually fall by 25% or more. This may still represent a similar percentage of the overall national health care budget, as total expenditures may be reduced for the same reasons. Alternatively, the health care budget will not change, as money saved on transplantation will be spent on other ailments.

Although organ transplantation accounts for a relatively small percentage of overall expenditures, it has been a particular target for insurance companies and other payors in view of the relatively large amount of money spent on each individual patient. At present, $5 billion is spent annually on only approximately 160,000 patients, who either receive an organ transplant during the year (currently about 20,000) or currently survive with a functioning organ transplant received in a previous year. This works out to approximately $31,000 per patient. The amount spent on the patient in the first post-transplant year, involving as it does the transplantation procedure itself, is of course substantially more than in subsequent years. For example, the approximate cost of a patient undergoing a heart transplant is $90,000 in the first year, but only $10,000 for subsequent years. For comparison, the average first-year costs for other organ transplants range from $45,000 for a kidney transplant to more than $125,000 for liver or lung transplants. It should be noted that the costs of organ transplants vary widely from country to country and are particularly expensive in the United States. In the United Kingdom, a kidney transplant has been estimated to cost only £10,000 to £15,000 (approximately $16,000–$23,000), with liver and heart transplants costing about £10,000 to £20,000.

There is also considerable variation between the costs at different transplant centers within the United States, ranging, for example, from less than $100,000 to more than $450,000 for a liver transplant (although actual reimbursement may be substantially less in many cases). It is this wide variation that forms the basis of many of the negotiations between insurance companies and transplant centers. If one center charges $100,000 for a transplant, and yet the center down the road or in the next city charges only $50,000, the insurer can threaten to send all of its transplant patients to the cheaper center (given comparable care and results). The "expensive" center will either have to cut its costs to become competitive or be squeezed out of the transplant business.

The same negotiations will clearly take place once xenotransplantation becomes clinically established. However, if prior experience with human donor organ transplantation is a guide, the insurance companies will refuse to cover the costs of a xenotransplant until it is a generally proven and established form of therapy. They deny payment for what are considered "experimental" or "investigational" forms of therapy, and take it on themselves to decide when a therapy can be considered established.

Roger Evans has drawn attention to the fact that organ transplantation attempts to treat "catastrophic diseases," and that all such diseases are expensive to treat. Indeed, the 13% of hospital patients in the United States with catastrophic diseases consume as much of the available resources as the remaining 87% of patients. Despite this expense, Evans, in his inimitable and slightly irreverent way, is at pains to point out that "the end of life can only be postponed." Taken to the extreme, he says, "the cost of dying now exceeds the expense of living."

Although the amount spent on the average transplant recipient is considerable—and is therefore singled out for special scrutiny by the health care financiers—it is not as high as that spent on many other patients (Table 16.1). For example, over $300,000 is spent on the care of a very premature baby

table 16.1

Estimated Cost of Treating Certain Conditions in the United States (in Dollars Per Patient)

	U.S. $
1. Premature baby during first year of life	300,000
2. Adolescent with major psychiatric disorder	200,000
3. Total intravenous nutrition	100,000
4. Severe burns	100,000
5. Bone marrow transplant	150,000
6. AIDS	40,000–140,000
7. Cancer	50,000
8. Maintenance hemodialysis	25,000–45,000

Data from P. Laing, *Sandoz—The Unrecognized Potential of Xenotransplantation,* Salomon Brothers, London, 1996; R. W. Evans, in *Xenograft 25,* M. A. Hardy (ed.), Elsevier, Amsterdam, 1989, p. 359; and R. W. Evans, personal communication, 1998.

during its first year of life. Nevertheless, organ transplants are among the most expensive medical treatments that can be offered to a patient.

Profits and Losses ○ ○ ○

The expenditure on any individual patient correlates closely with the condition of the patient at the time of the transplant. The sickest patients, particularly those on life support—for example, ventilators, cardiac assist devices, and so on—not only have the poorest post-transplant outcome but also accumulate the highest hospital charges, unless they die soon after the transplant. Xenotransplantation may have some beneficial impact on costs in this respect. With no restriction on the number of organs available, patients should be able to undergo organ transplantation electively when they are first deemed to need it. The all-too-frequent case of a patient clinging desperately to life while he or she awaits a donor organ will be a thing of the past. Not only should the post-transplant outcome be improved because the patient is in a better state to survive the procedure, but the post-transplant costs should be significantly reduced because the patient will recover more quickly and be able to leave hospital earlier.

The greatest financial saving, however, will be on the care of the patient *before* the transplant—an expense that is not normally taken into account. It is not uncommon for a patient awaiting a heart transplant to spend one or two months, or even longer, in an expensive intensive care unit, waiting precariously for a suitable donor organ to become available. As a stay in many intensive care units in the United States can amount to as much as $3,000 a day, the patient's hospital charges may easily exceed $150,000 before the transplant even takes place. We have personally known patients whose hospital bill exceeded $200,000 yet did not even survive to undergo a transplant. The loss of the patient's productivity in the community during this period is, of course, a further factor that is difficult to assess, but could be included as an indirect cost in the overall equation.

Long-term outpatient support will also no longer be essential while the patient awaits an organ. For example, chronic dialysis for kidney failure or drug therapy for advanced heart failure will be unnecessary. One of the standard forms of dialysis, hemodialysis, has a direct cost of up to $45,000 a year in the United States. By contrast, a kidney transplant currently costs approximately $45,000, and between $5,000 and $10,000 a year thereafter for anti-rejection therapy. Transplantation is estimated to produce a saving of nearly 60% when compared with lifelong dialysis. Clearly, there is a marked economic incentive in favor of a transplant, which also offers the renal failure patient a much better quality of life. Furthermore, the number of patients on chronic dialysis is continuing to rise. Without the advent of xenotransplantation, the annual cost of treating the world's pool of patients on dialysis—currently estimated to be 700,000 and costing $19 billion—is likely to grow steadily.

According to the Salomon Brothers report, about 20,000 admissions to U.S. hospitals each year are for patients who have fulminant hepatic failure. A two- or three-week stay in an intensive care unit for these patients while they await a suitable liver donor may at times result in a bill approaching $100,000. But these patients represent only a small percentage of the estimated 300,000 annual hospital admissions for less rapidly progressive liver failure. Although the cost of care of each of these less ill patients is less, it still amounts to a large amount of money. By enabling a liver transplant to be performed as soon as it is deemed necessary, xenotransplantation will eliminate many of these pretransplant expenses.

Because of the high incidence of heart disease in the Western world, the cost of maintaining patients in heart failure is extremely high. The American Heart Association estimates that there are approximately 3 million people with congestive heart failure in the United States. The combined total in the United States and Europe is estimated to be 6.8 million. Despite the adoption of preventive measures, both the incidence of congestive heart failure and its related mortality are increasing, presumably due to the aging of the population. In the United States, over 400,000 new patients with congestive heart failure are diagnosed every year, and there are about 250,000 deaths from this condition each year. It accounts for almost 1 million hospital admissions in the United States each year; in the United Kingdom, with a population of 59 million, the figure is about 125,000. Because of the poor prognosis and the need for hospitalization, congestive heart failure is an expensive condition to treat. The estimated annual treatment cost in the United States exceeds $10 billion. Even in the United Kingdom, where health care costs are generally considerably less than in the United States, expenditure on patients with heart failure approximates £500 million ($850 million). The social and economic cost of the loss of many of these patients from the workforce has also to be considered.

With the huge medical expenditure of maintaining patients with diabetes, and particularly of those with such economically debilitating diseases as Parkinson's and Alzheimer's, successful cell xenotransplants would certainly prove highly cost-effective.

The actual costs involved in a successful xenotransplant cannot yet be calculated, as the exact therapy that will be necessary has not been finalized.

If a transgenic pig organ is required, then the cost of the organ itself may be high. If tolerance to the graft can be achieved, the need for expensive long-term immunosuppressive drug therapy will be negated. Preventing the complications associated with such therapy will also greatly reduce the long-term costs of an organ transplant. But if we estimate for the sake of discussion that the cost of a xenotransplant will be comparable to that of a human organ today, then the amount spent on organ transplantation in the United States may well quadruple. A similar estimate has been made in the United Kingdom. In the United States, therefore, based on Roger Evans' "best guess," the total expenditure may increase from the current $5 billion to approximately $20 billion annually. This will represent more than 2% of total U.S. expenditure on health care. If a xenotransplant proves more expensive than an allograft, then the costs will increase accordingly. In a period of significant health care reform and budgetary reductions, not only in the United States but in most Western countries, this would appear to be a significant added burden to health care funding, unless offset by savings as outlined above.

There are those who believe that Roger Evans' best guess may be too conservative. The Salomon Brothers report estimates that the annual cost of carrying out kidney xenotransplants alone will be nearly $10 billion worldwide. Furthermore, if pig hearts become universally available, giving a transplanted heart to just those patients age 55 or below who are deemed in need of one would cost an additional $3 billion a year. This figure would increase to nearly $13 billion if those between the ages of 55 and 75 are included. These estimates are, of course, only intelligent guesses based on the data that are currently available. Nevertheless, since end-stage heart disease is so much more common than end-stage renal failure, expenditure on heart transplantation is likely to rise much more precipitously than that on kidney transplantation.

Handsome Rewards: The Impact of Xenotransplantation on the Pharmaceutical Industry ○ ○ ○

The Salomon Brothers report was primarily concerned with a review of the financial prospects for Sandoz, one of the major pharmaceutical companies involved in transplantation. (Since the 1996 report was issued, Sandoz has merged with another giant pharmaceutical company, Ciba-Geigy, to form a new company, called Novartis.) The report estimated that the immunosuppressive drug cyclosporine accounted for over 20% of Sandoz's pharmaceutical sales, with sales reaching over $1 billion per annum in the United States alone. It is a disproportionately profitable drug, accounting for an estimated

40% of Sandoz's pharmaceutical operating profit. From the perspective of the patient and the transplant surgeon, however, cyclosporine is worth every penny of its cost. Its introduction was a quantum leap in the care of organ transplant patients, and for many it has made the difference between life and death.

Unless immunological tolerance can be successfully induced—in which event the market for immunosuppressive drugs might collapse entirely—Salomon Brothers estimated that U.S. sales of cyclosporine would grow from $1 billion in 1994 to over $5 billion if xenotransplantation is successfully introduced. Perhaps it is therefore not surprising that, according to some reports, Novartis is spending an estimated $25 million a year on research in this field and is reputedly prepared to invest up to $1 billion in xenotransplantation technology. However, other factors may upset these calculations. First, the introduction of cheaper generic forms of cyclosporine by competitors of Novartis may alter the price-profit ratio. Second, new approaches to immunosuppression, such as the costimulatory blockade briefly mentioned in Chapter 6, may replace cyclosporine even for the treatment of patients with human organ transplants.

Organ transplantation is still, unfortunately, associated with many potential complications. The majority of these relate to the immunosuppressive drug therapy that the patient is required to take for the remainder of his or her life. To prevent or treat these complications, the patient is prescribed still more drugs. For example, steroid drugs can lead to gastritis and peptic ulceration, and so the patient may take daily antacids or drugs that reduce gastric acid secretion. Antibiotics may be prescribed to prevent certain infections that have a high incidence in immunosuppressed patients. These accessory drugs can double the patient's monthly drug bill. Indeed, the current overall expenditure on drugs for patients with organ transplants is estimated conservatively at $4 billion annually worldwide. So it is not only the pharmaceutical companies that manufacture immunosuppressive drugs that will profit from the introduction of xenotransplantation; many others will reap handsome rewards as well.

Conversely, companies that manufacture dialysis equipment or supplies are likely to be very adversely affected by the successful introduction of xenotransplantation. The unlimited supply of donor kidneys will inevitably reduce or even negate the need for long-term dialysis in many patients, who will be offered kidney transplantation at an early stage of their disease. Company income associated with dialysis will eventually fall to a small percentage of the present level, and in Western countries it could well disappear almost entirely.

How Much Is a Life Worth?
Can Society Afford Xenotransplantation? o o o

A full discussion of the ethics of health care—summed up by the Institute of Medicine report as "How much is saving a life worth?"—is beyond the confines of this volume. Society will nevertheless have to grapple with this question anew if xenotransplantation becomes a clinically feasible and successful form of therapy.

Most medical advances have initially proved expensive. As our experience grows, the costs have fallen dramatically. Open heart surgery is one such example; it was many times more expensive in its infancy 40 years ago than it is now. A second example is organ transplantation itself. The average hospital stay of a patient undergoing heart transplantation in 1980 was more than a month; in many centers today this has been reduced to less than 10 days, resulting in vast financial savings. Nevertheless, at least during the clinical development phase of xenotransplantation, allocation of scarce health care dollars may well result in less financial support for other, more mundane forms of therapy. Society must decide if it is willing to pay this price.

In practical terms, health care payors will probably await evidence that xenotransplantation is cost-effective, not only in comparison to allotransplantation but also in comparison with the continuing medical care of the transplant candidate. For example, when transplantation of a pig heart can be demonstrated to be less expensive than long-term drug therapy for heart failure *and* provide a better quality and length of life, then the payor will be prepared to foot the bill. Before this is clearly demonstrated, insurance companies and governments will be reluctant to pay for this form of therapy.

Many other factors will, of course, be considered in the equation whether to underwrite xenotransplantation. These include a consideration of possible alternative therapies—for example, the implantation of an artificial heart—and the financial pressures related to the demands of other patient groups not requiring transplantation. Premiums for health insurance may have to be raised to meet the added demands of xenotransplantation. The U.S. government will undoubtedly have to consider whether xenotransplantation will be covered by Medicare, as will governments of other countries with a socialized health care system, such as many of the European nations.

Should the community expend precious health care dollars and resources on a relatively small number of people? Ethicists Renee Fox and Judith Swazey have asked, "As poverty, homelessness, and lack of access to health care increase in our affluent country, is it justifiable for American society to be devoting so much of its intellectual energy and human and financial resources to the replacement of human organs?" Should there be a limit, for example, on the amount spent on transplantation or xenotransplantation? Should the public have a say in allocating funds for this type of expenditure? Dr. Alan Hull, former president of the National Kidney Foundation in the United States, has pointed out that there is no such limit or "say" with regard to other health care items, such as the amount spent on coronary artery bypass surgery, so why should there be one on transplantation? Roger Evans would suggest that if society is unable to afford transplantation services, then it would appear that it is unable to afford a wide range of other services as well.

This view may be appropriate when considering health care services as they are organized and financed in the United States, where individuals are free to purchase as much or as little health insurance coverage as they wish or can afford. To some extent, therefore, Americans really do get the health services they pay for. In countries where there is a national socialized health care system, such as the United Kingdom, the situation is rather more complex. All taxpayers contribute to the service, and therefore there is possibly more justification to put some limits to the service provided to the individual.

For example, should money be provided for a bone marrow transplant, estimated to cost in the region of $150,000, in a last, desperate effort to save the life of a patient with widespread cancer? Or on the even more expensive intensive care of premature infants? Should money be spent on the treatment of infertility when overpopulation exists in much of the world (and particularly when such treatment not infrequently results in multiple births)? In all of these discussions, it should be remembered that the cheapest form of care is to allow the patient to die.

What about preventive medicine? Wouldn't it be better to spend this money on preventing problems such as heart disease—encouraging people to improve their diets, get more exercise, have their cholesterol levels checked regularly, and so on? Or on reducing the incidence of liver disease by educating people on the detrimental effects of heavy alcohol intake? Or on reducing lung failure from emphysema or cancer by encouraging young people not to start smoking? Of course it would, if people would follow this advice. But, just as there is a problem with noncompliance in patients with organ transplants, so are large sections of the public notoriously resistant to (or incapable of) doing what they know would be in the best interests of their health. Lung cancer, for example, would essentially be abolished if no one smoked; a lethal disease would be almost eradicated overnight. Preventive medicine, when it depends largely on the individual's willpower and discipline, has failed miserably. In all probability, no amount of money would enable preventive measures to be fully successful. Furthermore, Roger Evans is of the opinion that few studies have demonstrated the cost-effectiveness of measures aimed at prevention. Too often, for example, screening for diseases is applied indiscriminately, resulting in an attenuation of anticipated cost savings.

In answering the objection that xenotransplantation will cause social injustice by lavishing expensive medical resources on relatively few people, possibly at the expense of basic care for the many, Harold Vanderpool points out that one interpretation of the concept of "justice" holds that "unusual benefits should be given to people with unusual needs."

The U.K. "Blueprint" o o o

One sensible approach would be similar to that followed in the United Kingdom for heart transplantation. Initially, only three centers were funded by the government health service to perform the procedures. These national centers drew patients from throughout the country. This not only controlled expenditure until the therapy became fully established, but also ensured that the transplants were performed solely in institutions with adequate facilities and where increasing experience and expertise could be concentrated. As heart transplantation became more established and the results steadily improved, a larger number of centers was opened, each of which took responsibility for offering the service to a particular region of the country. This eliminated the need for patients to travel great distances for the service. So successful was this policy that the report of the Nuffield Council on Bioethics recommended that this should be the preferred method of introducing xenotransplantation into the U.K. health service.

This system could theoretically provide a blueprint for introducing xenotransplantation into other countries. However, although it works well in a country with a government-funded, centrally controlled health care system, it may not be possible to introduce it so successfully in a country such as the United States, where most health care is funded by private insurance companies and where transplantation is carried out in independent, largely autonomous medical centers. In the United States, a government restriction preventing a center from performing xenotransplants may well be met by loud outcries, including complaints of restriction of practice and charges that such a policy effectively limits this form of therapy to various patient groups. However, although normally it might be exceedingly difficult for the U.S. government to control the introduction of a new form of therapy in this way, it might be successful with regard to xenotransplantation. The necessity to monitor patients for infection will enable government agencies to have far more control over xenotransplantation than over many other procedures—at least until it is an established form of therapy. Even then, it is likely that insurance companies may be able to control the expansion of the therapy by agreeing to pay for xenotransplantation only at carefully chosen centers that have demonstrated a real interest and expertise in this field.

The Direct Costs of Organ Transplantation o o o

There are three major costs with regard to allotransplantation: the cost of the care of the donor and the organization of donor organ retrieval, the cost of the transplant operation itself, and the long-term care of the transplant patient, which primarily relates to the cost of immunosuppressive and other drug therapy.

When a human organ is donated, there are, of course, no direct costs for the organ itself. In most Western countries, the donor's family does not receive any form of financial reward or compensation. Indeed, in many countries it is illegal for them to be offered any financial reimbursement whatsoever—not even a few coins to make a telephone call or buy a cup of coffee. However, the expense of monitoring and preparing a potential human donor in the hospital before the organs are excised is considerable. In addition, the indirect administrative costs of the regional organ procurement organization (OPO), whose staff organize the care of the donor and coordinate organ retrieval, have to be factored into the financial equation.

Maintenance after a potential donor has been identified involves care of the brain-dead body in an intensive care unit for several hours, sometimes for a day or more. This is highly labor-intensive, and may involve the full-time attention of both an intensive care unit nurse and the transplant coordinator. Numerous blood tests are performed to exclude infection, investigations such as echocardiography to monitor heart function are routinely carried out, and sometimes expensive investigations such as coronary arteriography (X-ray examination of the arteries of the heart) are required. These add up to considerable expenditure, which is ultimately passed on to the patients who receive the various donor organs.

These costs relating to the care of the donor will be negated by the introduction of xenotransplantation. Although the organs may be expensive, the pig donor will require no such intensive care. Nor will multiple surgical teams be required to hire expensive private jets to descend on the donor center in the middle of the night. In the United States, these various donor-related costs (excluding transport of the surgical teams, which can be as much as $5,000 for each team) vary from a minimum of about $7,500 for a kidney retrieval to as much as $25,000 at some centers for retrieval of organs such as the lung or liver. The local OPO in whose region the donor hospital is geographically situated passes on these costs to the recipients of the organs by billing the transplant centers where the transplants are to be performed.

These costs vary considerably from OPO to OPO. Although the OPO works as a nonprofit organization—that is to say, no shareholders receive any share of the profits relating from its work—there appears to be no legal restriction on what the OPO can charge for the organs. If the OPO finds itself barely covering its costs (direct and indirect) after the payment of salaries and other expenses, it can unilaterally elect to increase its charges for organs during the following year. This may seem appropriate, but the system can be abused. For example, the OPO board of directors (which is usually made up of local transplant surgeons plus a few members of the public) may decide to pay the executive director and other staff particularly generously, or to allow other perks or expenses. (We know of one small OPO where the executive director is reimbursed approximately twice as well as comparable administrators with equal or greater responsibility at nearby hospitals, and better than the state governor and even the local college football coach.) Such indirect expenditure can, of course, greatly increase the cost of the organs. The only real brake on what an OPO can charge comes from the health care payors (mostly the insurance companies and the government), which have begun to set limits on what they will reimburse for the various organs. The OPO, therefore, like the transplant center, frequently does not get reimbursed the full amount of what it charges.

How Much Is a Pig Worth? o o o

The above human-donor-related expenses will be replaced by the cost of purchasing a suitable pig organ. This charge will clearly reflect the cost of research that has led to the development of the pig, particularly if it is transgenic, as well as the cost of ensuring that the pig herd is free of infectious disease and microorganisms that could be transferred to the patient. By the time the costs of removing and transporting the organ to the transplant hospital are factored in, we suspect that the overall costs may be rather higher than those relating to human organs today. As the breeding and rearing of the donor pigs will almost certainly be a commercial enterprise, even in countries with socialized health care systems, the organs will likely become cheaper as the enterprise grows and more and more organs are utilized, and especially when there are several suppliers of such pigs.

The Salomon Brothers report assumed that one donor animal would be required for each organ used (although it is more likely that several organs will be removed from each donor pig). They estimated, therefore, that some 50,000 transgenic pigs would be required worldwide each year just to fulfill present requirements. The capital costs of setting up multiple pig-breeding units to provide these pigs is estimated to be $500 million, including the cost of the land, and the annual operating expenses might be as much as $30 million. Even if an average of five organs are obtained from each pig, the capital and maintenance costs will be significant. If xenotransplantation becomes fully established for both cell and organ transplants, the ultimate projected annual need for porcine donors might increase to almost 500,000.

The Salomon Brothers report estimated that the cost of each organ to the transplant center would be about $12,000, which is comparable to the average cost of obtaining a human donor organ in the United States. It is more likely that a company breeding specialized pigs will price them significantly higher, particularly if they are transgenic and if the company has a monopoly on such pigs. After retrieval and placement of the heart, liver, both kidneys, and both lungs from one individual human donor, a local OPO may pass on costs (to the respective transplant centers) that total in the region of $75,000. In view of the great advantage of their immediate availability, the suppliers may aim to achieve a significantly higher income from the multiple organs obtained from one individual pig.

New Expenditures ○ ○ ○

New expenditures will come in countries where allotransplantation is rarely performed at present, and from the introduction of cell transplants that have proved hitherto impossible.

The economic impact of xenotransplantation will clearly be felt most in countries such as Japan, where the transplantation of human cadaveric organs is not culturally accepted today. (Japanese transplant surgeons believe that xenotransplantation will be more acceptable to the country's population.) Current expenditures on organ transplantation in Japan are minimal when considered as a proportion of the health care budget: only about 400 organ transplants (mainly from living, related donors) are performed in that country annually. This can be compared with the current (and totally inadequate) 3,500 per year in the United Kingdom, which has only half the population of Japan. If xenotransplantation is successfully introduced in Japan, the number of transplants there could increase between 35 and 70 times.

Although the cost of retrieving pancreatic islet cells from the three to eight pigs that it is estimated will be needed to treat each diabetic patient would be high, the ability of xenotransplanted cells to prevent the many late and debilitating complications of this disease would more than prove its economic benefit. For example, a diabetic patient may develop kidney failure, requiring dialysis or a kidney transplant, or develop obstruction to blood flow in the arteries of the legs, necessitating vascular reconstructive surgery. Such complications can clearly be a major expense. Diabetes affects an estimated 15 million patients in the United States, of whom at least 2 million require insulin therapy. The initial worldwide market for islet cell transplants could, therefore, be on the order of 4 million patients.

The cost of the introduction of new forms of therapy, such as pig brain tissue transplants into patients with degenerative diseases, including Parkinson's or even Alzheimer's disease, is difficult to estimate. However, the current cost of these diseases to the community in terms of the loss of productive members of society and/or the need for institutional or home nursing or other care, although difficult to quantify accurately, is immense. (In these terms, Alzheimer's disease alone is estimated to cost nearly $100 billion in the United States annually.) If xenotransplantation eventually offers a cure— or at least delays the onset of such conditions—then it would prove hugely cost-effective.

"Rationing" of Health Care o o o

There is already rationing of health care in most countries, including the United States. Many in the United States, not least among the medical profession, are quick to denigrate socialized systems of health care, such as Britain's. The criticism is frequently made that such socialized systems provide inadequate service. Certainly, unless urgent treatment is essential, treatment is "rationed" by the establishment of a long waiting list of those requiring any given therapeutic option (for example, hip replacement surgery for arthritis). Only by restricting nonurgent services to a certain number of patients each year can costs be controlled. In defense of such systems, though, it can at least be argued that in the United Kingdom no one is prevented from being considered for therapy or from being put on the waiting list purely as a result of his or her inability to pay. In the United States, where over 40 million people have no health insurance whatsoever, a patient who does not have personal wealth or adequate insurance is unlikely even to make it to the waiting list for a heart or liver transplant at most centers. Let us not fool ourselves: rationing is very real on financial grounds in most, if not all, of the world's health care systems, including that of the United States. Xenotransplantation will not change this situation, but the limitation provided by an insufficient number of donor organs will no longer serve as a "natural" rationing process.

Market-Driven or Government-Controlled? ○ ○ ○

In view of the chronic shortage of human donor organs, the Organ Procurement and Transplant Network (OPTN), administered by the United Network for Organ Sharing (UNOS), was set up in the United States in the mid-1980s to regulate their allocation and distribution. Whether UNOS has been successful in achieving its goal of an equitable and efficient distribution of the organs that become available remains controversial. Most European countries have centralized systems that play a similar role, either nationally or even internationally.

Successful xenotransplantation would eliminate the shortage of organs and thus the need for a central service that matches available organs to recipients. This raises the possibility of a commercialized decentralized organ supply system where the transplant center can purchase animal organs directly from the supplier. The elimination of intermediate parties such as UNOS, whose administrative expenses are considerable, would reduce costs in terms of both time and money. Any further role for a centralized service like UNOS may well be limited to monitoring the national registry of xenotransplant recipients to assess the success of xenotransplantation. The tracking of potential transmission of infectious diseases is likely to be carried out by other government agencies with expertise in this field, such as the Centers for Disease Control.

Sanders Chae, whose review of the legal implications of xenotransplantation was referred to in Chapter 15, points out that this fundamental change in organ supply raises difficult philosophical and political questions. A commercialized market system raises the potential for a variable price structure on donor organs. All organs would have to satisfy designated governmental (FDA and PHS) requirements in order to minimize the possibility of transmitting infectious disease, but, within the range of acceptability, the best quality animal organs may command the steepest prices, while organs that are sufficient but in some way less ideal may be available at lower prices. For example, some transgenic pig organs (like some drugs) may be shown to be rather more successful than others at helping to avoid rejection, although both may be satisfactory enough to have gained FDA approval. The producers of the better pigs may, not unreasonably, choose to price their organs higher than those of their competitors.

As a consequence of this, the ability to pay might determine the quality of the organ that a patient receives. Wealthy patients, or those with the best health insurance, would receive the best animal organs, while others might have to settle for organs that are less optimal. The question is whether society is willing to accept a system that exposes desperately ill patients to market forces. In reality, this restriction is not so very different from the present system in the United States, where a patient without health insurance or substantial personal financial means is frequently precluded from undergoing organ transplantation or, indeed, many other medical procedures.

In the United States, the alternative would be congressional action to maintain a centralized system by integrating xenotransplantation into the current system. Although there would be no shortage of organs, UNOS would continue to distribute them, though the basis on which it would do so is hard to determine. Presumably, as UNOS would have a monopoly on the transplant business, it might have some control over the pricing of the donor organs. However, any system that attempted to establish a fixed price for organs would, by eliminating much of the profit motive, risk undermining the market forces that would encourage organ suppliers to generate better animal organs.

In summary, the introduction of xenotransplantation into the care of patients with terminal organ failure will have major repercussions on the cost of transplant services in all developed countries. Although there will be significant savings in some areas, the overall impact of xenotransplantation will be to increase health care expenditure. As with all other innovations that come with a price, society will have to decide whether it wishes to accept this added financial burden for the sake of those who will benefit.

chapter 17

A Vision with a Task

The Model T Pig ○ ○ ○

Whenever the first clinical trial of xenotransplantation using pig organs is initiated, the surgical team will undoubtedly be embarking upon this undertaking with relatively primitive technology. The results will probably be only modest, if that, but the experience gained will allow sequential improvements to be made until the results will match and eventually surpass those of human organ transplantation today. It would be unduly optimistic to expect the first patients who receive xenotransplants to do as well as those currently receiving human organ transplants. The more pertinent question is whether they will do better *with* a xenograft than *without* one. For these patients, the alternative to an animal organ will not be a human one, which for one reason or another will already have been ruled out, but rather conventional medical therapy. Clearly, no one wants a pig organ that functions for only one month, but there would be a period of time—if the quality of life was good—that would have made the procedure worthwhile.

No matter how advanced the technology, however, there will always be those who caution against such a trial. But, as David White has pointed out, you cannot wait until you know you can swim before being allowed in the water. Or, to quote him again, "We are talking about designing a Model T Ford, while other people are saying, 'Let's not go out driving until we have a Ferrari.'"

Those who preach against moving ahead with xenotransplantation draw attention to the potential risks of rejection, infection, the development of tumors, and the other side effects of immunosuppressive drug therapy, and suggest that it is not ethical to subject a patient to these several risks and unknowns. Jeff Platt and others have reminded us that these identical concerns were being raised only 20 or 30 years ago with regard to the use of *human* organs for transplantation. They applied equally to allotransplantation then as they do to xenotransplantation today. If bold surgeons and brave patients had not been prepared to face those unknowns and challenges not that many years ago, the many hundreds of thousands of patients who have benefited from organ transplantation worldwide since that time would not have done so. There comes a time when, in the words of medical ethicists Renee Fox and Judith Swazey, both patients and surgeons have to have "the courage to fail." Without this courage, no real progress will be made.

In Oklahoma, home to many Native Americans, there is a saying: "Timing has a lot to do with the success of a rain dance." One has to have one eye on the Weather Channel, or at least on the clouds, before beginning the dance. As far as xenotransplantation is concerned, the forecast is encouraging. The technology is developing fast, and if it is not quite ready for us to perform our "dance" yet, it should be soon.

We may then be in a position to resolve some of the ethical dilemmas generated by the use of human organs. We will no longer have to be concerned with transplanting a substandard donor organ. Decline in organ quality is sometimes the result of the changes that take place in the body during the agonal period as the potential donor develops brain death. When we were in Cape Town, our group was among the first to document these changes. With xenotransplants, the source pig will be a healthy anesthetized animal, and injury caused by brain death will no longer be a factor. Every transplant surgeon has been faced with the agonizing decision of whether or not to use a less-than-ideal donor organ in a patient who desperately needs a transplant. The donor pig organ will be known to be perfect. If for any reason it is not, it can be discarded and another chosen.

No longer will we be forced to use an organ from a donor that we know harbors the hepatitis virus, cytomegalovirus, or another potentially serious microorganism. The pig organ will be known to be free of such infectious organisms.

Today, one kidney is transplanted into every renal transplant patient, but there is evidence that two kidneys might survive longer than one. Instead of an average of 10 years' function, as is achieved by the single transplanted kidney, the greater functioning capacity of two kidneys might sustain the patient for many years longer. After all, we are each born with two kidneys, not one. Such is the shortage of human donor organs that surgeons can allocate only one to each patient. It would be easy, however, to allocate two pig kidneys to every patient.

The Advance of Science ○ ○ ○

We are today experiencing the greatest biological revolution the world has ever known. With the quite amazing advances taking place—seemingly almost on a weekly basis—the remaining hurdles of xenotransplantation will undoubtedly be overcome. Xenotransplantation will be established as an important therapy for thousands of patients, in many of whom it will prove lifesaving. And yet, to put this whole endeavor into the perspective of the long-term progress of medical science, xenotransplantation will almost certainly be only a transitory therapeutic option. It will bud, flower, and wither, to be superseded by yet other medical advances that will negate its benefits. Diabetes may be corrected by gene therapy in infancy. Heart disease may be prevented by knowledge of how atherosclerosis develops. Kidney failure may be treated by cloning new human kidneys from the patient's own kidney cells or by developing a new kidney from a human stem cell. A new human liver may be constructed from a few healthy liver cells using tissue engineering techniques. The advance of science is seemingly inexorable.

Which of the current methodologies will enable xenotransplantation to be fully successful? Which of the above—or other—techniques will lead to therapies or preventions that make xenotransplantation obsolete, like so many therapies physicians have advocated and administered in the past? As Shakespeare wrote in *Macbeth:*

> *If you can look into the seeds of time,*
> *And say which grain will grow and which will not,*
> *Speak.*

But for the present, and certainly well into the 21st century, the scientists and surgeons earnestly struggling to solve the remaining problems of xenotransplantation are among the most fortunate of people. In the words of an unknown writer:

> *A vision without a task is a dream.*
> *A task without a vision is drudgery.*
> *A vision with a task is the hope of the world.*

Xenotransplantation researchers are indeed fortunate to have both a vision and a task.

appendix

Key steps in developing guidelines on xenotransplantation

1. August 1993: Ethics Committee of the Transplantation Society, "Human Xenotransplantation" (position paper published in the *Transplantation Society Bulletin*, 1, 8, 1993).

2. January 1995: Nuffield Council on Bioethics (United Kingdom), *Animal-to-human Transplants: The Ethics of Xenotransplantation* (report published in London, 1996).

3. June 1995: Institute of Medicine (United States), *Xenotransplantation—Science, Ethics and Public Policy* (report published by the National Academy Press, Washington, DC, 1996).

4. March 1996: Organization for Economic Cooperation and Development (OECD), *Advances in Transplantation Biotechnology: Animal to Human Organ Transplants (Xenotransplantation)* (report published in Paris, 1996).

5. August 1996: U.K. Advisory Group on the Ethics of Xenotransplantation (Kennedy Report), *Animal Tissues into Humans* (published by Her Majesty's Stationery Office, Norwich, 1997).

6. September 1996: U.S. Department of Health and Human Services, Public Health Service, "Draft Guidelines on Infectious Disease Issues in Xenotransplantation" (*Federal Register*, Vol. 61, No. 185, pp. 49920–49932).

7. January 1997: U.K. Xenotransplantation Interim Regulatory Authority set up (interim until National Standing Committee on Xenotransplantation is set up).

8. September 1997: Council of Europe recommendation on xenotransplantation.

9. December 1997: Ethics Committee of the Transplantation Society, "The Transplantation Society and Xenotransplantation (Draft Guidelines)" (published in the *Transplantation Society Bulletin*, 6, 11–14, 1997).

10. December 1997: Food and Drug Administration Center for Biologics (CBER) Xenotransplantation Advisory Subcommittee to examine ongoing clinical trials.

11. 1997: World Health Organization, *Draft Recommendations on Xenotransplantation and Infectious Disease Prevention and Management* (prepared by the Division of

Emerging and Other Communicable Disease Surveillance and Control), WHO, Geneva, 1997).

12. January 1998: U.S. Department of Health and Human Services public forum, Washington, DC, "Developing U.S. Public Health Policy in Xenotransplantation," proposal by U.S. Public Health Service for National Xenotransplantation Advisory Committee.

13. March 1998: Joint Organization for Economic Co-operation and Development (OECD)/New York Academy of Sciences workshop, "International Issues in Transplantation Biotechnology, Including the Use of Non-human Cells, Tissue and Organs," New York (published as "Xenotransplantation: Scientific Frontiers and Public Policy," *Annals of the New York Academy of Sciences*, 862, 1998).

14. July 1998: U.K. Department of Health—Health Service Circular HSC 1998/126, *Clinical Procedures Involving Xenotransplantation* (this includes the United Kingdom Xenotransplantation Interim Regulatory Authority, *Guidance on Making Proposals to Conduct Xenotransplantation on Human Subjects*).

15. March 1999: U.S. Department of Health and Human Services, *Guidance for Industry: Public Health Issues Posed by the Use of Nonhuman Primate Xenografts in Humans.*

16. March 1999: Organisation for Economic Co-operation and Development (OECD), *Xenotransplantation: International Policy Issues.*

17. 1999: Joint Council of the American Society of Transplantation and the American Society of Transplant Surgeons. *Position Paper on the Initiation of Clinical Trials of Xenotransplantation.*

glossary of selected biomedical terms

This section has been compiled in part from several sources, including some of the references listed in the Bibliography.

Acute cellular rejection An immunological process that occurs within a few days, weeks, or months following *organ* or *tissue transplantation*. It is mainly caused by the action of a group of *white blood cells*—the *T cells*—acting against the grafted tissue.

Acute vascular rejection An immunological process which occurs when foreign *antigens*, such as those expressed on the *endothelium* of a xenotransplanted organ, stimulate the production of *antibodies* in the recipient. There may also be additional activity associated with various groups of recipient *white blood cells*. This process causes rejection within days or weeks. (See also *hyperacute rejection*.)

AIDS (acquired immunodeficiency syndrome) Disease caused by the human immunodeficiency virus (HIV), which infects a type of *white blood cell* called *T cells*, and thus destroys the patient's cell-mediated immune response. This leaves the individual susceptible to a variety of opportunistic diseases, particularly certain infections and cancers.

Allograft (Allotransplant) The *tissue* or *organ* that has been transplanted from one individual to another genetically different member of the same *species*. An example would be a kidney transplanted from one human to another.

Allotransplantation The transplantation of *organs* or *tissues* between genetically different members of the same *species*.

Antibodies *Immunoglobulin* proteins produced by *B cells* in response to stimulation by an *antigen*. Antibodies circulate in the blood and bind to specific antigens on the *cells* of invading *microorganisms* or of transplanted *tissues*. Antibodies can activate *complement* and destroy the foreign cells directly, or they can stimulate *white blood cells* to carry out the destruction.

Antigens Molecule that is capable of inducing an *immune response*, such as the production of *antibodies* or the activation of the host *T cells*. This generally occurs only if the antigen is recognized as foreign by the *immune system*. Infectious *organisms* entering the body, such as *bacteria* or *viruses*, have antigens on their surface. When the antigens are recognized as foreign, an immune response is mounted to protect the body from infection. An immune response is also induced by the antigens on the cells of a transplanted organ or tissues.

B cells (B lymphocytes)   *White blood cells* that produce *antibodies*. They are an important element of the *immune response*.

Bacteria (*sing.* bacterium)   Any of a group of single-celled *microorganisms*. Some are capable of causing diseases in humans and animals.

Bovine   Relating to cattle.

Brain death   Occurs when a person has irreversibly lost all brain function, including the capacity for consciousness and the capacity to breathe. The state of brain death represents the point at which a person is accepted as being dead even though his or her heart is still beating. The diagnosis of brain death is required before *cadaveric organs* can be removed for transplantation.

Cadaveric organs   *Organs* for transplantation obtained from individuals who have died.

Cardiac   Relating to the heart.

Cell   The smallest component of the living *organism* capable of carrying out essential life processes, such as the ability to grow, reproduce, and respond to stimuli.

Chimerism   A state in which two (or more) genetically different populations of cells coexist. A chimeric animal is the product of two (or more) different sets of parents (i.e., two independent conceptions).

Chronic rejection   An immunological process that usually occurs many months or years after *transplantation*, and results in a deterioration in function of the transplanted *organ*. The immune mechanisms are poorly understood, but are thought to involve *antibodies* and cellular (including *T cell*) mechanisms.

Clones   A number of identical *organisms* (or *cells*) of like genetic constitution that are derived by asexual *replication* of a single original individual cell. Clones may be obtained from a single embryonic, fetal, or mature adult cell.

Cloning   See *nuclear transfer*.

Complement   A group of some 30 *plasma* proteins that participate in various *immune responses* usually activated by an appropriate *antibody*. When activated, they interact in sequence, leading to the immune destruction of invading *microorganisms* (e.g., *bacteria*) or a transplanted *organ* or *tissues*, such as an organ *xenograft*.

Complement activation   The initial triggering of the *complement* cascade. *Antigen-antibody* complexes act as the trigger.

Complement-regulatory proteins (regulators of complement activity)   A group of molecules found on the surface of the body's *cells* that prevent *complement* from attacking the body's own *tissues*. Complement regulatory proteins are species-specific, and check or down-regulate the complement cascade to prevent unnecessary damage being done to the body's own tissues. Examples include decay accelerating factor (DAF), cluster of differentiation 59 (CD59), and membrane cofactor protein (MCP). *Transgenic* animals can be genetically modified to express a complement regulatory protein from a different species.

Concordant   Indicates a closely related *species*.

DNA (deoxyribonucleic acid)   A molecule found principally in the *nucleus* of the *cell*. It bears the coded genetic information required to determine the structure and function of an *organism*.

Dialysis   System used to treat patients with kidney failure (who may be waiting for a kidney transplant) whereby toxic substances are removed from the blood.

Discordant   Indicates a distantly related *species*.

Dopamine   A chemical found in the brain and other *tissues*. There is good evidence that dopamine deficiency is one of the causative factors in *Parkinson's disease*.

ELAD   *Extracorporeal* liver assist device (artificial liver).

Endogenous retroviruses   *Retroviruses* are *viruses* that infect *cells* and then become inserted into the genetic material (*genome*) of the cells. Endogenous retroviruses are the result of retroviral infection of germline cells (egg or sperm) and are passed from parent to offspring in a Mendelian manner. Although they usually remain in a dormant state in the natural host, the transplantation of an *organ* from one *species* (e.g., pig) to another (e.g., human) might reactivate them, leading to the production of new retroviruses, which could cause illness.

Endothelial cells (endothelium)   *Cells* that form the lining of blood vessels and certain other structures.

Epitope   An *antigen* on the surface of a *cell*.

Extracorporeal support   A method of partially taking over the function of a failing *organ* by passing the patient's blood through a substitute organ placed outside the body. For example, whole pig livers or liver assist devices (ELADs) containing pig hepatocytes have been used to temporarily support patients with liver failure.

Fungus (*pl.* fungi)   Any of a diverse group of single or multicellular *microorganisms*. Some fungi can cause disease in humans and animals.

Gal epitope   A sugar *antigen* (galactose-α1, 3-galactose) present on the surface of the cells of lower mammalian *species*, including the pig. The antigen is recognized as foreign by human *xenoreactive antibodies*. The Gal epitope is a sugar molecule found on the surface of pig cells. When pig organs are transplanted into humans, Gal acts as an antigen. It is recognized by human antibodies and *hyperacute rejection* is triggered.

Gene   Unit or region of *DNA* that contains the hereditary information needed to carry out a specific function, for example, the synthesis of a particular protein. Broadly, one gene encodes one protein.

Gene therapy   The introduction of a *gene* into the body's *cells*, usually in an attempt to alleviate disease.

Genetic modification/manipulation   The process by which the *DNA* of an *organism* is changed by artificial means.

Genome   Term used to describe all of the genetic material in the *nucleus* of a cell. (Some *microorganisms* do not have nuclei, but do have genomes.)

Germ line   Pertaining to the *cells* from which eggs or sperm are derived. These cells contain *DNA* that will be inherited by offspring.

Hemophilia   An inherited blood clotting disorder which results in prolonged bleeding even after minor injury.

Hepatic   Relating to the liver.

Higher primates   Category that includes such primate species as humans and apes.

Human immunodeficiency virus (HIV)   See *AIDS*.

Humoral   Relates to any process involving circulating *antibodies*.

Hyperacute rejection   The most rapid form of transplant rejection. It occurs between *discordant species* because of the effect of *xenoreactive natural antibodies* in the recipient's blood. In hyperacute rejection, host blood clots throughout the donor organ within minutes, causing dramatic failure of the organ. All or most natural *antibodies* reacting against pig *antigens* recognize a sugar antigen termed the *Gal epitope*.

Immune response   A selective response mounted by the *immune system* of humans and animals. Specific *antibodies* and/or *T cells* are produced against invading *microorganisms*, transplanted *tissues*, and other material recognized as foreign.

Immune system   Collectively, the *cells* and *tissues* that enable animals to mount a specific protective *immune response* to invading *microorganisms*, transplanted tissues, and other material recognized as foreign to the body.

Immunodeficiency state   A deficiency of the *immune response*, involving *humoral* (antibody-mediated) and/or cell-mediated (including *T cells*) *immunity*, as in *AIDS*.

Immunoisolation   The separation of transplanted *tissue* from the *immune system* of the host by an artificial barrier.

Immunological response   See *immune response*.

Immunological tolerance   The acceptance of a transplanted *organ* (i.e., without rejection) without continuing immunosuppressive drug therapy.

Immunologist   Expert or student of the immune system.

Immunology   Science of the *immune system*.

Immunosuppression The use of drugs or other agents to suppress the *immune system*. Immunosuppressive drugs are taken by transplant recipients to prevent *organ* or *tissue rejection*.

Islets (islets of Langerhans) Groups of *cells* scattered throughout the pancreas that secrete insulin and other hormones involved in regulating blood sugar levels. Destruction of the insulin-producing cells of the islets results in type I diabetes. These clusters of cells in the pancreas were first described by the German pathologist Paul Langerhans in 1869, although he had no idea what their function might be.

Microorganism A minute or microscopic living *organism*, including *bacteria, viruses* and *fungi*. Some are capable of causing disease in humans and animals.

Mutation The process during which the *DNA* of an *organism* changes or mutates. In *viruses* and other infectious organisms, mutations can lead to the emergence of organisms with new characteristics. In some cases they may be more infectious, or cause more serious disease.

Neurological Relating to the nervous system (brain, spinal cord, nerves).

Neurotrophic factors A class of compounds that can promote the survival, growth, or repair of nerves whose degeneration leads to a number of serious *neurological* disorders, including Alzheimer's disease, amyotrophic lateral sclerosis (Lou Gehrig's disease), and Huntington's disease.

Nuclear transfer (cloning) Process (which was used to create Dolly the sheep) that involves removing the *nucleus* of an egg and replacing it with the nucleus of another *cell*. The cell is then stimulated to grow and proliferate and, under certain ideal conditions, can develop to form a whole viable *organism* or animal. This animal would be a *clone* of the original animal from which the cell nucleus was derived.

Nucleus (*pl.* nuclei) The part of a *cell* that contains the chromosomes, which are essential to the transmission of hereditary character.

Organ A collection of different *tissues* that form a distinct structural and functional entity in the body. Examples of solid organs include liver, heart, brain, and kidney.

Organism Any living thing, which may be an animal, a plant, or certain *microorganisms*.

Pathogen An infectious agent (often a *microorganism)* that is capable of causing disease.

Perfusion The transfer of fluid (such as blood) through a *tissue* or an *organ*.

Plasma The fluid part of blood. Plasma differs from *serum* in containing the precursors of important substances involved in blood clotting (in addition to the other constituents of serum).

Plasma cells Mature *B cells*.

Porcine Relating to pigs.

Prion A form of *protein* that is thought to cause a type of disease called spongiform encephalopathy. Examples are, in cattle, bovine spongiform encephalopathy (BSE) or "mad cow disease," and, in humans, Creutzfeldt-Jakob disease. The diseases lead to degeneration of the brain and spinal cord. Prions are unusual because they appear to be a unique example of an infectious agent that does not contain genetic material.

Recombination   A form of *mutation* in which two *organisms* (e.g., *viruses*) exchange genetic material, resulting in the production of a new organism, which may have different characteristics.

Rejection   See *transplant rejection.*

Renal   Relating to the kidney.

Respiratory   Pertaining to breathing.

Retrovirus   A family of *viruses* with a special replication mechanism that includes incorporation of genetic material into the *DNA* of the *organism* it has infected. Examples of retroviruses include the human immunodeficiency virus (HIV), which causes *AIDS*, and certain tumor-causing viruses. See also *endogenous retrovirus.*

RNA (ribonucleic acid)   Is similar to *DNA* in structure, but performs a different function in living *cells*. RNA is used to translate genetic information into proteins. Some viruses (e.g., HIV) contain RNA but not DNA.

Serum   The fluid component of clotted blood that contains *antibodies* and other soluble material. See also *plasma.*

Source animal   The "donor" animal from which *tissues* and *organs* are taken.

Species   A group of *organisms* that have similar characteristics and are capable of interbreeding to produce offspring.

Specific- (or defined-) pathogen-free (SPF)   The term given to animals that have been bred in captivity and isolated from other animals in order to avoid infection by excluding specific known *pathogens*. The animals are kept in conditions that reduce the risk associated with contracting these infectious agents. No contact is allowed with non-SPF animals.

T cells (T lymphocytes)   *White blood cells* (derived from the thymus gland) of the *immune system* that interact to produce the cellular *immune response.*

Tissue   An organized aggregate of similar *cells* that perform a particular function (e.g., bone marrow, nerve tissue). Different tissues may group together to form an *organ.*

Tolerance   See *immunological tolerance.*

Transgene   A *gene* that an *organism* would not normally have in the *genome* of its *cells*. The gene might have been purposely transferred from one *species* to another.

Transgenic   Term used to describe an *organism* that, through *genetic modification*, has a heritable foreign *gene* (known as a *transgene*) incorporated into the *genome* of each *cell.*

Transplant rejection   The process where the host *immune response* recognizes the transplanted *organ* or *tissue* as foreign and acts against it, leading to damage or destruction of the organ or tissue. See also *hyperacute, acute vascular, acute cellular,* and *chronic* rejection.

Transplantation   The removal of *organs, tissues,* or *cells* from one *organism* (such as a human body) and their implantation into another.

Vascular   Pertaining to blood vessels, including arteries, capillaries and veins.

Viable   Capable of living. This will apply to *organs,* most *tissues,* and *cells* that may be transplanted, but does not include, for example, sterilized bone, which is nonviable (dead).

Virus   Any of a vast group of minute infectious *microorganisms* composed of a sheath of protein encasing a core of *DNA* or *RNA.* A virus is not normally considered to be a living organism since it cannot live independently. Instead, viruses must infect living *cells* and reproduce inside them.

White blood cells   Blood *cells* that do not contain hemoglobin (which is the pigment in the red blood cells). They include *T cells* and *B cells,* which are involved in the body's immune response.

Xenograft (xenotransplant)   The *tissue* or *organ* that has been transplanted from a member of one *species* to a member of another *species.* An example would be a transplanted pig kidney in a baboon or human.

Xenosis (*pl.* xenoses)   See *xenozoonosis.*

Xenotransplantation   The *transplantation* of an *organ* or *tissue* between members of different *species.*

Xenozoonosis (*pl.* xenozoonoses)   A *zoonosis* that can be transmitted by the *xenotransplantation* of animal *tissues* or *organs.*

Zoonosis (*pl.* zoonoses)   Any infectious disease that can be transmitted by the transfer of an infectious *microorganism* (or *pathogen*) from an animal to a human.

bibliography

Advisory Group on the Ethics of Xenotransplantation (UK). *Animal Tissue into Humans*. Norwich: Her Majesty's Stationery Office, 1997.

Bach, F. H., Fishman, J. A., Daniels, N., et al. Uncertainty in xenotransplantation: Individual benefit versus collective risk. *Nature Medicine*, 4, 141–144, 1998.

Brent, L. *A History of Transplantation Immunology*. San Diego, London: Academic Press, 1997.

Cohen, L. R. *Increasing the Supply of Transplant Organs: The Virtues of an Options Market*. Austin: R. G. Landes, 1995.

Cooper, D. K. C., Kemp, E., Platt, J. L., White, D. J. G. (eds). *Xenotransplantation*. (Second edition.) Heidelberg: Springer, 1997.

Cooper, D. K. C., Kemp, E., Reemtsma, K., White, D. J. G. (eds.). *Xenotransplantation*. (First edition.) Heidelberg: Springer, 1991.

Daar, A. S. Ethics of xenotransplantation: Animal issues, consent and likely transformation of transplant ethics. *World Journal of Surgery*, 21, 975–982, 1997.

——— Xenotransplantation and religion: The major monotheistic religions. *Xeno*, 2, 61–64, 1994.

Dixon, P. *The Genetic Revolution*. Kingsway America, 1993.

Fishman, J. A., Sachs, D. H., Shaikh, R. (eds.). *Xenotransplantation—Scientific Frontiers and Public Policy*. Annals of the New York Academy of Sciences, volume 862, 1998.

Fox, R. C., Swazey, J. P. *The Courage to Fail*. Chicago: University of Chicago Press, 1974.

Hardy, M. A. (ed.). *Xenograft 25*. Amsterdam: Elsevier Science, 1989.

Health Council of the Netherlands; Committee on Xenotransplantation. *Xenotransplantation*. Publication 1998/01E. Rijswijk: Health Council of the Netherlands, 1998.

Institute of Medicine (U.S.). *Xenotransplantation: Science, Ethics and Public Policy*. Washington, DC: National Academy Press, 1996.

Kuss, R., Bourget, P. *An Illustrated History of Organ Transplantation—The Great Adventure of the Century*. Rueil-Malmaison: Sandoz, 1992.

Laing, P. *Sandoz—The Unrecognized Potential of Xenotransplantation*. London: Salomon Brothers, 1996.

Land, W., Dosseter, J. B. (eds.). *Organ Replacement Therapy: Ethics, Justice, Commerce*. Berlin: Springer, 1991.

Lanza, R. P., Langer, R., Chick, W. L. (eds.). *Principles of Tissue Engineering*. San Diego: Academic Press, 1997.

—— *Yearbook of Cell and Tissue Transplantation, 1996/97*. Dordrecht: Kluwer, 1996.

Moller, G. (ed.). Xenotransplantation. *Immunological Reviews*, 141, 1–276, 1994.

National Kidney Foundation. *Public and Professional Attitudes towards Xenotransplantation and Other Options to Increase Organ Availability*. Southeastern Institute of Research, Richmond, Virginia: April, 1998.

Nuffield Council on Bioethics (U.K.). *Animal-to-Human Transplants: The Ethics of Xenotransplantation*. London, 1996.

Organization for Economic Co-operation and Development (OECD). *Xenotransplantation: International Policy Issues*. March, 1999.

Prentice, E. D., Fox, I. J., Dixon, R. S., Antonson, D. L., Lawson, T. L. History, donor considerations and ethics of xenotransplantation and xenoperfusion. In: *Research Animal Anesthesia, Analgesia and Surgery*. Proceedings of a conference sponsored by the Scientists Center for Animal Welfare (SCAW). September 1994, pp. 25–36.

Real, J. *Serge Voronoff and Mathieu Jaboulay*. Paris: Communauté Européene et Abbeville Press, 1997.

Regan, T. *The Case for Animal Rights*. Los Angeles: University of California Press, 1983.

Remensnyder, J., et al. *Report of the Xenotransplantation Advisory Committee* of the Massachusetts General Hospital, Boston, 1997.

Ronchi, E. (Biotechnology Unit, Organization for Economic Cooperation and Development [OECD]). *Advances in Transplantation Biotechnology: Animal to Human Organ Transplants (Xenotransplantation)*. OCDE/GD(96)167. Paris: OECD, 1996.

Singer, P. *Animal Liberation*. New York: Random House, 1975.

U.K. Department of Health. *Clinical Procedures Involving Xenotransplantation*. (Circular HSC 1998/126). Includes UKXIRA *Guidance on Making Proposals to Conduct Xenotransplantation on Human Subjects*. 1998.

U.S. Department of Health and Human Services Public Health Service. *Biological Response Modifiers Advisory Committee: Xenotransplantation Subcommittee Meeting*, December, 1997 (meeting transcript can be obtained from the FDA home page: http://www.fda.gov).

—— *Developing U.S. Public Health Policy in Xenotransplantation*, January, 1998 (meeting transcript can be obtained from the FDA home page: http://www.fda.gov).

—— *Draft Guidelines on Infectious Disease Issues in Xenotransplantation*. Federal Register 61, 185, 49920–49932, 1996 (document can be obtained from the FDA home page: http://www.fda.gov).

—— *Guidance for Human Somatic Cell Therapy and Gene Therapy*, March, 1998 (updates and replaces the 1991 *Points to Consider*) (document can be obtained from the FDA Home Page: http://www.fda.gov).

—— *Guidance for Industry: Public Health Issues Posed by the Use of Nonhuman Primate Xenografts in Humans*. Federal Register 64, 65, 16743–16744, 1999. (Document can be obtained from the FDA home page: http://www.fda.gov).

—— *Proposed Approach to Regulation of Cellular and Tissue-Based Products*, February, 1997 (document can be obtained from the FDA home page: http://www.fda.gov).

Vanderpool, H. Y. Critical ethical issues in clinical trials with xenotransplants. *Lancet,* 351, 1347–1350, 1998.

Voronoff, S. *Rejuvenation by Grafting.* New York: Adelphi, 1922.

Weiss, R. Transgenic pigs and virus adaptation. *Nature,* 391, 327–329, 1998.

Witt, C. J., Meslin, F.-X., Heymann, D. (Division of Emerging and Other Communicable Disease Surveillance and Control [EMC]). *Draft World Health Organization Recommendations on Xenotransplantation and Infectious Disease Prevention and Management.* Geneva: WHO, 1997.

World Medical Association Declaration of Helsinki. *Recommendations Guiding Physicians in Biomedical Research Involving Human Subjects.* London: World Medical Association, 1964 (amended 1975, 1983, 1989, 1996).

Youngner, S. J., Fox, R. C., O'Connell, L. J. (eds.). *Organ Transplantation: Meanings and Realities.* Madison: University of Wisconsin Press, 1996.

index